Health Policy Developments

Issue 5

Reinhard Busse, Annette Zentner,
Sophia Schlette (eds.)

Health Policy Developments

Issue 5
Focus on Public-Private Mix, Patient Safety,
Public Health

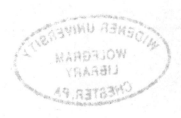

| Verlag Bertelsmann**Stiftung**

Bibliographic information published by Die Deutsche Bibliothek

Die Deutsche Bibliothek lists this publication in the
Deutsche Nationalbibliografie; detailed bibliographic data
is available on the Internet at http://dnb.ddb.de.

© 2006 Verlag Bertelsmann Stiftung, Gütersloh
Responsible: Sophia Schlette
Copy editor: David L. Hopper
Production editor: Sabine Reimann
Cover design: Nadine Humann
Cover illustration: Aperto AG, Berlin
Typesetting: digitron GmbH, Bielefeld
Printing: Hans Kock Buch- und Offsetdruck GmbH, Bielefeld
ISBN-10: 3-89204-873-8
ISBN-13: 978-3-89204-873-2

www.bertelsmann-stiftung.de/publications

Contents

Introduction

The Bertelsmann Stiftung has a tradition of comparative policy research and international benchmarking. It has established a reputation for providing sound advice and innovative problem-solving in the field of economic and social politics.

The International Reform Monitor (www.reformmonitor.org), initiated in 1999 and now in its sixth year, is one example of this benchmark expertise. It primarily covers social and labor market issues. An example of the Foundation's expertise in comparative health policy research is "Reformen im Gesundheitswesen" (Esche, Böcken and Butzlaff (eds.) 2000), a study that compared health policy reforms in eight countries.

The success of both projects underscored the need and the potential demand for timely and regular information on health policy issues in countries with similar socioeconomic patterns. To this end, the Foundation established a separate monitoring tool, the International Network for Health Policy and Reform.

The International Network for Health Policy and Reform

Since 2002, the International Network for Health Policy and Reform has brought together health policy experts from 20 countries around the world to report on current health reform issues and health policy developments in their respective countries, 17 of which are covered in this issue. Geared toward implementation, the Network aims to narrow the gap between research and policy, providing timely information on what works and what does not in health policy reform.

Participating countries were chosen from a German perspective. We specifically looked for countries with reform experience relevant for Germany.

Partner institutions were selected taking into account their expertise in health policy and management, health economics or public health. Our network is interdisciplinary; our experts are economists, political scientists, physicians or lawyers. Many of them have considerable experience as policy advisers, others in international comparative research.

Australia	Centre for Health Economics, Research and Evaluation (CHERE), University of Technology Sydney
Austria	Institute for Advanced Studies (IHS), Vienna
Canada	Canadian Policy Research Networks (CPRN), Ottawa
Denmark	Institute of Public Health, Health Economics, University of Southern Denmark, Odense
Estonia	PRAXIS, Center for Policy Studies, Tallinn
Finland	STAKES, National Research and Development Center for Welfare and Health, Helsinki
France	IRDES, Institut de Recherche et de Documentation en Economie de la Santé, Paris
Germany	Bertelsmann Stiftung, Gütersloh Department of Health Care Management, Berlin University of Technology (TUB)
Israel	The Myers-JDC-Brookdale Institute, Smokler Center for Health Policy Research, Jerusalem
Japan	National Institute of Population and Social Security Research (IPSS), Tokyo
Netherlands	Institute of Health Policy and Management (iBMG), Erasmus University Rotterdam
New Zealand	Centre for Health Services Research and Policy, University of Auckland
Poland	Institute of Public Health, Jagiellonian University, Krakow
Singapore	Department of Community, Occupational and Family Medicine, National University of Singapore (NUS)

Slovenia	Institute of Public Health of the Republic of Slovenia, Ljubljana
South Korea	School of Public Health, Seoul National University
Spain	Research Centre for Economy and Health (Centre de Recerca en Economia i Salut, CRES), University Pompeu Fabra, Barcelona
Switzerland	Institute of Microeconomics and Public Finance (MecoP), Università della Svizzera Italiana, Lugano
UK	LSE Health & Social Care, London School of Economics and Political Science (LSE)
USA	The Commonwealth Fund, New York Institute for Global Health (IGH), University of California Berkeley/San Francisco

Survey preparation and proceedings

Issues were jointly selected for reporting based on what the network partners identified as the most pressing issues for reform. Subsequently, the issues were arranged into clusters:
- Sustainable financing of health care systems (funding and pooling of funds, remuneration and paying providers)
- Human resources
- Quality issues
- Benefit basket and priority setting
- Access
- Responsiveness and empowerment of patients
- Political context, decentralization and public administration
- Health system organization/integration across sectors
- Long-term care
- Role of private sector
- New technology
- Pharmaceutical policy
- Prevention
- Public health

If an issue did not fit into one of the clusters, participants could create an additional category to report the topic.

Reporting criteria

For each survey, partner institutes select up to five health policy issues according to the following criteria:
- Relevance and scope
- Impact on status quo
- Degree of innovation (measured against national and international standards)
- Media coverage/Public attention

For each issue, partner institutions fill out a questionnaire aimed at describing and analyzing the dynamics or processes of the idea or policy under review. At the end of the questionnaire, our correspondents give their opinion regarding the expected outcome of the reported policy. Finally, they rate the policy in terms of system dependency/transferability of a reform approach.

The process stage of a health policy development is illustrated with an arrow showing the phase(s) a reform is in. A policy or idea does not necessarily have to evolve step by step. Also, depending on the dynamics of discussion in a given situation, a health policy issue may well pass through several stages during the time observed:

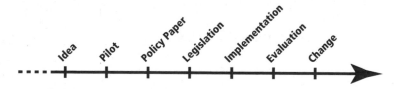

Idea refers to new and newly raised approaches voiced or discussed in different forums. Idea could also mean "early stage": any idea present but not anywhere near formal inception. In this way, a "stock of health policy ideas in development" is established, permitting the observation of ideas appearing and disappearing through time and "space."

Pilot characterizes any innovation or model experiment implemented at a local or institutional level.

Policy Paper means any formal written statement or policy paper short of a draft bill. Included under this heading is also the

10

growing acceptance of an idea within a relevant professional community.

Legislation covers all steps of the legislative process, from the formal introduction of a bill to parliamentary hearings, the activities of driving forces, the influence of professional lobbyists and the effective enactment or rejection of the proposal.

Implementation: This stage is about all measures taken towards legal and professional implementation and adoption of a policy. Implementation does not necessarily result from legislation; it may also follow the evidence of best practices tried out in pilot projects.

Evaluation refers to all health policy issues scrutinized for their impact during the period observed. Any review mechanism, internal or external, mid-term or final, is reported under this heading.

Change may be a result of evaluation or abandonment of development.

Policy ratings

A second figure is used to give the reader an indication of the character of the policy. For this purpose, three criteria are shown: public visibility, impact and transferability.

Public Visibility refers to the public awareness and discussion of the reform, as demonstrated by media coverage or public hearings. The ratings range from "very low" (on the left) to "very high" (on the right).

Impact: Ranging from "marginal" (on the left) to "fundamental" (on the right), this rating criterion illustrates the structural or systemic scope and relevance of a reform, given the country's current health care system.

Transferability: This rating indicates whether a reform approach could be adapted to other health care systems. Our experts assess the degree to which a policy or reform is strongly context-dependent (on the left) to neutral with regard to a specific system, that is, transferable (on the right).

The figure below illustrates a policy that scores low on visibility and impact but average on transferability.

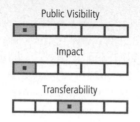

Public Visibility

Impact

Transferability

Project management

The Bertelsmann Stiftung's Health Program organizes and implements the half-yearly surveys. The Department of Health Care Management, Berlin University of Technology (TU Berlin), assisted with the development of the semi-standardized questionnaire. We owe special thanks to Ines Galla in the Bertelsmann Stiftung for managerial and editorial support.

The results from the fifth biannual survey, covering the period from November 2004 to April 2005, are presented in this book. Out of 62 reported reforms, 28 were selected.

While we describe current developments from the reporting period in detail on our Web site, we chose a somewhat different approach for presenting the findings in this report. Criteria for selection were scope, continuity and presence in public debate during and beyond the reporting period proper. With this in mind, we looked at topics from the first four surveys independently of their present stage of development or implementation.

This fifth issue of "Health Policy Developments" pays special attention to four concurrent health policy topics, all of them high on health policy agendas in a variety of developed countries:
- Public-private mix
- Patient safety
- Public health
- Pharmaceutical policy and drug evaluation

In line with the Health Policy Network's news and monitoring function, the last chapter, "Newsflash," reports on policies to improve end-of-life care in Israel, on recent developments to increase transparency of hospital bills in Singapore, and on proposals to promote research in primary health care centers in Finland.

Reports from the previous four and the fifth survey round can be looked up and researched on the network's Web site, www.healthpolicymonitor.org. Both those reports and this publication draw upon the partner institutions' reports and do not necessarily reflect the Bertelsmann Stiftung's point of view.

Thanks of course go to all authors from our partner institutions and to those who helped as reviewers and proofreaders.

Authors: Rob Anderson, Michael O. Appel, Toni Ashton, Alek Aviram, Gabi Ben Nun, Netta Bentur, Frankki Bevins, Shuli Brammli-Greenberg, David Cantarero (Universidad de Cantabria), Karine Chevreul, Terkel Christiansen, Luca Crivelli, André den Exter, Kees van Gool, Revital Gross, Marion Haas, Sebastian Hesse, Jos Holland, Sirpa-Liisa Hovi, Phuong Trang Huynh, Annakaisa Iivari, Neva Kaye (National Academy for State Health Policy), Ilmo Keskimäki, Reuven Kogan, Soonman Kwon, Marjukka Mäkelä, Esther Martínez García, Tom McIntosh, Carol Medlin, Lim Meng Kin, Julien Mousqués, Anja Noro, Adam Oliver, Zeynep Or, Valérie Paris, Dominique Polton, Jaume Puig-Junoy, Bruce Rosen, Masayo Sato, Christoffer Tigerstedt, Renée Torgerson, Lauri Vuorenkoski, Sarah Weston und Jonathan Wittenberg.

Reviewers/proofreaders: Anne-Marie Audet, Celia Bohannon, Iva Bolgiani, Jennifer Edwards, Mary Ries.

Comments and suggestions to the editors on this fifth half-yearly report are more than welcome. This series will continue to evolve, change, and, as we hope, improve. That is why any input will be helpful.

Reinhard Busse
Annette Zentner
Sophia Schlette

Public-private mix

For decades, there have been controversial debates among health policy makers about the balance between state and market, between regulation and competition. Many countries are attempting to find compromise solutions to these disputes that combine private entrepreneurship with the role of the state in the implementation of health policies and public health programs.

Behind the buzzword of privatization, however, lies neither a uniform strategy nor a uniform trend. Privatization includes altered financing models with more self-participation and/or a larger private insurance market, as well as changes in the ownership of hospitals or the public contracting of private service providers.

The conflict about the appropriateness of the public-private mix is encountered in all developed countries. It reflects power relationships and conflicts of interest just as much as differing ideologies and diverging expectations about the potential of the two concepts.

Privatization in health care has many meanings

Some associate "state" with bureaucracy and inefficiency and "market" with efficiency and innovation; they argue that public regulation should be limited to a minimum. Others view public regulation as positive; they maintain that competition and deregulation reduce quality, increase costs and cause social inequalities. In the opinion of market skeptics, privatization inevitably leads to an erosion of access to health care, above all for groups of the population who are particularly at risk. The case reports in this chapter on reforms in the United States (see page 16), France (see pages 27 and 30) and Switzerland (see page 18) illustrate aspects of this debate.

In the field of conflict between the differing goals of a health care system—improved health, public satisfaction, a fair distribution of burdens, and high efficiency—it is to be expected that the debate about the "right mix" between public and private will remain just as controversial in future.

Sources and further reading:
Busse, Reinhard, Jonas Schreyögg and Christian Gericke. Health Financing Challenges in High Income Countries. HNP Discussion Paper Series. Washington, D.C.: World Bank 2006 (in press).
Maynard, Alan (ed.). *The public-private mix for health.* Abingdon: Radcliffe Press 2005.
Maarse, Hans (ed.). *Privatisation in European Health Care. A comparative analysis in eight countries.* Maarssen: Elsevier Gezondheidszorg 2004.

United States: Individual mandate for health insurance

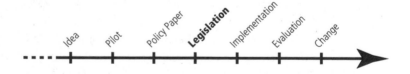

Public Visibility

Impact

Transferability

Health insurance to become mandatory

California is undertaking another attempt to pass legislation on mandatory health insurance coverage. Since the referendum in November 2004 (accepted with the slimmest of margins) freed employers from the obligation to provide health insurance coverage for employees (see issues 2 and 3 of "Health Policy Developments"), every citizen is now to be given an individual mandate.

According to a proposal submitted jointly by Democrats and Republicans in February 2005, all Californians will have to provide proof with their tax declaration that they and their dependents have health insurance coverage through their employer, a state health insurance program or private insurance. Otherwise they will automatically be included in a regional public health insurance program and the premium will be charged against their income tax, for example by being deducted from any tax refund that is due.

In a time of polarization in U.S. politics, such a bipartisan initiative is unusual. However, in the opinion of experts such as the Institute of Global Health, the proposed legislation has little chance of being passed. Many Californian politicians, particularly Democrats, think that the draft has not been properly thought through. They are not confident that the goal of universal health insurance coverage can be achieved without provisions to include, for example, those who do not submit tax returns (such as students, illegal immigrants and people with low incomes). Proposal, still vague, lacks support

But elsewhere, too, the proposal meets with little support. Civil rights groups object that the policy would criminalize the 6.4 million Californians who currently lack insurance. Though these include people with low incomes, the needy and the elderly, the largest subgroup (42 percent) are people 18 to 34 years old who are not insured through their employer, through state programs or privately. Civil activists are worried that individuals will find themselves in a very weak negotiating position with respect to the insurance companies and will be unable to obtain suitable and affordable coverage. The legislation offers only very vague framework conditions, such as that there should be first-dollar coverage for medically indicated preventive care and a maximum annual deductible of $5,000 (€4,100) for all other care.

The health insurance companies have also declared that they will resist the initiative. In order to support those with low incomes who cannot afford health insurance, the legislative initiative proposes that the state should levy a gross premium tax on health care services plans which are currently exempted from this tax. The employers also risk losing a tax privilege: Companies will only be able to set off payments for health insurance premiums up to a certain limit for taxation purposes. However, if an employer takes out insurance for particularly needy employees (i.e., those earning less than 50 percent of the poverty level), the state provides subsidies.

The Californian proposal is the first serious attempt nationwide to legislate an individual mandate for health insurance, though this model has been discussed from time to time in other

17

U.S.-wide trend:
Shifting the health
risk to the
individual

states. The Californian approach is in line with the policies of the Bush administration, which has proclaimed the need for more individual responsibility. A prime example of the strategy adopted by the Republicans at the national level is the heavily promoted "medical savings account"—a tax-exempt personal savings account from which medical costs can be paid. The common feature of all those approaches is that instead of the community or the government, the individual is given responsibility for health care and the possible financial risk for illness.

> *Sources and further reading:*
> Nation, Joe, and Keith Richman. A Bipartisan Solution to Comprehensive Healthcare Reform. http://republican.as sembly.ca.gov/pdf/RichmanHealthcare0205.pdf.

Switzerland: A drop of solidarity in the ocean of inequality

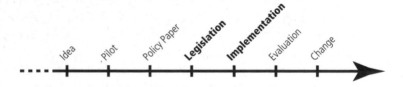

Public Visibility

Impact

Transferability

As of January 2007, Swiss families with low and medium incomes will pay only half the health insurance premium for their children.

The legislation passed in March 2005 by the Swiss parliament marks the end of a lengthy reform process aimed at easing the burden on families and lower-income earners under the Swiss per-capita premium system. However, it did not achieve the original goals of unifying the various systems of premium reductions in the 26 cantons and making real progress in redressing the social inequality of health care financing.

Since 1996, health insurance premiums in Switzerland have been the same for all those insured in a particular fund, irrespective of age, household income and the individual risk of illness. Although the benefit basket is identical, the premium depends on the costs of care at the place of residence and varies considerably among the competing health insurance funds. The tax-funded subsidies provided for lower-income households and for families vary widely from canton to canton. Thus, in 2003, a four-person family with a gross annual income of €45,000 paid on average 1.5 percent of available income for subsidized health insurance premiums in the canton of Wallis, compared with 14 percent in the canton of Geneva. Since rising expenditures in the health care system have meant that the per-capita premiums have increased continuously in recent years, the Swiss middle class has come to complain of the considerable financial burden of health insurance contributions.

Individual premiums impact on the middle class

In light of the discussion in Germany and elsewhere regarding funding options for health care systems, the reform process in Switzerland is particularly fascinating. Swiss experts note that in times of steadily rising health care expenditures on the one hand and increasing budget deficits in the public sector on the other, it can be extremely difficult to work against the undesirable effects of a per-capita premium system in the context of a federal state.

Learning from Switzerland

Not only was the so-called social goal abandoned, under which Swiss citizens who paid more than 8 percent of their annual taxable income for health insurance fund premiums were entitled to state support. A second proposal prepared by a parliamentarian commission and taken on by the Federal Council a few months later was not successful either. Even more ambitious from the viewpoint of equity, it aimed at making the level of premium subsidy dependent on income in five regressive steps. The proposal failed twice—in December 2003 it was rejected by parliament, and in the April 2004, under the influence of the cantons on the hearings, this proposal was strongly modified until it took the shape of the actual solution (for the second revision of the Health Insurance Act, see issues 2 and 3 of "Health Policy Developments").

Social goals not achieved

Not surprisingly, the cantons are among the core opponents of a uniform income limit for claims to premium subsidy. According to estimates, the number of those entitled to a subsidy would increase drastically, and the financial burden on the cantons would increase by 7.2 percent annually. Currently, the cantons

Cantons refuse to accept role of financial losers

only pay about one third of the support from their own budgets; the remaining two thirds are funded by transfer payments from the central government. In 2004, these amounted to CHF 2 billion (€1.3 billion), increasing at an annual rate of 1.5 percent. But the burden sharing between the cantons and the federal government is currently under discussion. According to proposals, the national contribution to premium subsidies would be frozen at a maximum of 25 percent of health care expenditures for 30 percent of the population from 2008 on. The new allocation system would thus leave it to the cantons to make good any financial shortfalls from budgets.

Solidarity:
Between young
and old or
between rich and
poor?

In June 2004, the Swiss Conference of Cantonal Directors of Public Health presented its own counter-proposal: Solely children should be freed from premiums, and young adults under 25 years should pay half the premium. It was argued that this would establish greater solidarity between young and old. But the proposal did not find a sufficient majority in parliament, in part because richer and poorer families would have profited equally and thus there would have been no redistribution between the rich and the poor.

Another proposal in September 2004 from the ranks of the Christian Democrats attempted to combine the models of the Federal Council and the cantons but also failed to find a majority. According to this idea, families with low incomes (i.e., up to four times the minimum state pension) would pay no premium for their children, and families with a medium income (up to six times the minimum state pension) would pay only half the premium for their children.

Least common
denominator

After three years of debate, there were signs at the end of 2004 that a compromise would be reached between the cantons and the federal government for the regulation of premiums. Since the income limits are not longer specified in the legislation, the cantons felt that their constitutional right of autonomy in social affairs was sufficiently respected. In the current version, the cantons have a free hand to determine the limits for low or medium incomes below which premium subsidy will be provided for children. They also determine whether to use the federal taxable income, the cantonal taxable income or the net income after tax as the basis for claims. Finally, they themselves can determine the level of premium subsidy for children, which can be 50, 60 or 70 percent.

The premium reduction systems of some cantons already meet the requirements of this legislation, but the budgets for other cantons are under considerable financial pressure. It is to be feared that the regulations will continue to differ considerably from canton to canton. In terms of vertical and territorial equity, the Swiss reform is therefore a drop in the ocean. It does not represent a breakthrough for the country either in terms of family policies or in terms of social policies. Switzerland, one of the richest industrial nations, will continue to have a health care system with one of the lowest levels of financial equity in Western Europe.

Lowest equity level in Western Europe

Sources and further reading:
Balthasar, Andreas, Oliver Bieri, and Fransiska Müller. Monitoring 2004. Die sozialpolitische Wirksamkeit der Prämienverbilligung in den Kantonen. Swiss Federal Office of Public Health 2005. www.bag.admin.ch/kv/forschung/d/2005/Monitoring_2005_d.pdf (summary in English).

Bundesamt für Gesundheit. Statistik der obligatorischen Krankenversicherung 2003. www.bag.admin.ch/kv/statistik/d/2005/KV_2003_DE_v030205.pdf (in German).

Dürr, Markus. Für die Abschaffung der Kinderprämien. Entlastung der Familien—administrative Vereinfachung. *Neue Zürcher Zeitung,* October 28, 2004 (in German).

Nationalrat. Bundesgesetz über die Krankenversicherung. Teilrevision. Prämienverbilligung. Debate on March 3, 2005. www.parlament.ch/ab/frameset/d/n/4707/119514/d%5F n%5F 4707 %5F11 951 4%5 F1195 15. htm (in German and French).

Schweizerischer Bundesrat. Botschaft zur Änderung des Bundesgesetzes über die Krankenversicherung (Prämien verbilligung) und zum Bundesbeschluss über die Bundesbeiträge in der Krankenversicherung. www.admin.ch/ch/d/ff/2004/4327.pdf (in German).

Ständerat. Bundesgesetz über die Krankenversicherung. Teilrevision. Prämienverbilligung. Debate on December

12, 2004. www.parlament.ch/ab/frameset/d/s/4706/11694
3/d_s_4706_116943_116968.htm (in German and French).
Wagstaff, Adam, et al. Equity in the finance of health care:
some further international comparisons. *Journal of Health
Economics* (18) 1999: 263–290.

Germany: Co-payments for outpatient care

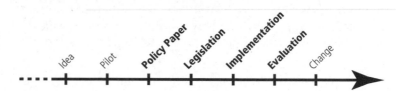

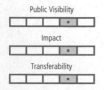

According to the Gesundheitsmonitor (Health Monitor) 2005, a
survey from the Bertelsmann Stiftung interviewing a representative panel of 1000 insurees twice a year, the introduction of
co-payments for outpatient visits in Germany in January 2004 has
reduced the number of consultations made, as was intended.
However, unwanted effects have also been observed; for example,
lower-income patients in relatively poor health have avoided visiting a physician.

User fees for office visits were introduced as part of the Statutory Health Insurance Modernization Act of 2004. This comprehensive health care reform was negotiated between the government (Social Democrats and Greens) and the main opposition
party (Christian Democrats). One of its central goals was to contain costs in the German health care system.

Several countries have introduced user fees to shift the financial burden to the patient and discourage unnecessary outpatient
visits (Donaldson and Gerard 2004). User fees especially aim to
reduce office visits for minor illnesses.

Germans see their doctor more often than other Europeans

In Germany, physician claims data for 2000 show that patients
with statutory insurance saw a physician at least 7.8 times on
average per year. This figure is lower than actual outpatient visits
because it documents only the first visit per quarter; all subsequent visits to the same physician are not reflected in the claims

data. According to various surveys, the number of actual outpatient visits to physicians has increased in the past decade. Between 1999 and 2002, the average rate of visits to office-based physicians was reported at 9.5 to 11.5 per year, varying by survey. International comparisons indicate that Germany thus has a higher number of outpatient contacts per person and year than the average of 6.2 for the 15 western EU member states.

One problem with user fees is that it is difficult to say whether the visits avoided were unnecessary or necessary. Another possible phenomenon is that patients forego seeing a physician in an early stage of a disease and wait until treatment becomes inevitable. This translates into even more office visits and treatment, putting an even higher financial burden on the system. To a certain extent, user fees shift the decision of whether a disease is severe or not from the physician to the patient.

While there may not have been much disagreement among politicians about introducing user fees, the same cannot be said of the other stakeholders involved. Such stakeholders include some policy makers and other interest groups within the system, such as patient representatives and consumer advocacy organizations. Criticism has focused on the social aspect of user fees.

Before this reform, Germany was one of the few countries without any kind of co-payments or user fees in the ambulatory care sector. Under the legislation that took effect in January 2004, an adult must pay €10 for the first office visit to a general practitioner or specialist in ambulatory care in each calendar quarter. This user fee covers additional visits within that quarter to that physician and to others, typically specialists, if referred by the physician first consulted. A patient who sees another physician in the same quarter without a referral must pay another €10 user fee.

The reform additionally increased co-payments for inpatient care and for pharmaceuticals. In an attempt to limit the financial burden for patients, the overall ceiling for cost sharing was newly defined: No one pays more than 2 percent of his or her annual gross income; the chronically ill and those on social security do not pay more than 1 percent of their annual gross income.

Ceiling for cost-sharing

Furthermore, there are several exemptions to the co-payment rules:

- Children under 18 are excluded from co-payments.
- All preventive medical checkups are excluded.
- Prenatal checkups for pregnant women are excluded.

To analyze changes in physician contacts, we must first distinguish between two ways of looking at outpatient visits. One way is to ask whether the overall number of patients visiting a physician (cases) went down. The second is to ask whether individual patients went to see a physician less often.

Results from the Gesundheitsmonitor 2005 survey show the following:
- After the reform, the overall number of office visits decreased and the number of referrals increased.
- The number of insurees who did not see any physician decreased between spring 2003 and spring 2005.
- The overall number of patient visits (cases) remained more or less constant. However, the number of specialist visits decreased. Patient visits in primary care did not decrease.
- The number of office visits per patient, the more meaningful figure overall, decreased by 8 percent in the time between spring 2003 and spring 2005. The physician group most affected was internal specialists and general practitioners.

This is actually in line with the well-known moral hazard theory, which states that patients avoid physician visits to save costs. Surprisingly, the number of those patients who saw their physician more than 10 times a year decreased, while the number of patients who saw their physician four to five times a year increased. This goes against the moral hazard theory. One would expect "high users" not to react because they are likely to see a physician every quarter anyway and cannot save any money by reducing visits. Those with few visits should show stronger reactions. One would expect them to reconsider a visit or postpone it until the beginning of the next quarter.

Did co-payments lead patients to do without important office visits?

According to the moral hazard theory, important outpatient visits have a very low elasticity of demand; that is, they are not postponed or avoided because of user fees.

The Gesundheitsmonitor asked: "How would you describe your health status?" and "Do you suffer from a chronic disease for which you see a physician at least once in a quarter and have to take medication on a regular basis?" These questions were combined with other questions regarding the number of outpatient visits before and after the introduction of co-payments. Data from the Gesundheitsmonitor show a drop in the number of outpatient visits for the group of patients who judged their own health as poor. From 2003 to 2005, the average number of office visits in this group decreased from 23 to 16 visits per year. Between 15 and 20 percent in the group with poor health made fewer visits.

Both results suggest that patients in relatively poor health visited a physician less often after the user fee was introduced. However, it cannot be said whether patients avoided only unnecessary visits or important ones as well. The survey responses indicate that an overall reduction carries the risk that patients might also avoid important physician visits. However, this inference is not based on empirical data analysis.

According to the moral hazard theory, user fees should lead to a fairly strong reduction in visits in low-income groups. As mentioned above, the legislation introduced a ceiling pegged to annual gross income. No one is expected to pay more than 1 percent of his or her gross income (1 percent for the chronically ill and the least well off). Despite this, results from the Gesundheitsmonitor found the highest proportion of patients foregoing an outpatient visit within the lowest income group (37 percent compared to the average of 28 percent). Higher-income groups showed the greatest tendency to postpone their visits.

Did reactions differ by income groups?

Interestingly, the reduction was highest in the population under age 35. This finding shows that older patients are not reacting as much to the reform as much as younger patients.

In summary, the introduction of user fees for outpatient visits in Germany clearly has reduced the number of office visits. However, unwanted effects can also be observed; for example, patients in relatively poor health made fewer visits to a physician. In addition, low-income groups have a higher rate of avoidance than the higher income groups. Unfortunately, the Gesundheitsmonitor data do not allow a distinction between necessary and unnecessary visits, but the overall number of reduced visits indicates that some patients made do without important visits.

Finally, the Gesundheitsmonitor findings do not entirely support the moral hazard theory. The data imply that the avoidance of outpatient visits is not entirely related to income, because the groups that earned less than €500 per month show the same effect as groups earning between €3,000 and €5,000 per month.

Hence the user fee has a social effect and critical aspects from a medical perspective that should be carefully scrutinized over time. Furthermore, it can be stated that the policy instruments introduced to make the user fees more socially adjusted are not as equitable as they were intended to be.

Sources and further reading:

Donaldson, Cam, and Karen Gerard. *Economics of health care financing: The visible hand.* Houndmillis: Palgrave Mcmillan 2004.

Gebhardt, Birte. Zwischen Steuerungswirkung und Sozialverträglichkeit – eine Zwischenbilanz zur Praxisgebühr aus Sicht der Versicherten. *Gesundheitsmonitor 2005. Die ambulante Versorgung aus Sicht von Bevölkerung und Ärzteschaft.* Jan Böcken et al. (eds.). Gütersloh: Verlag Bertelsmann Stiftung, 2005 (in German).

Glossary on the German health care reform: Das Glossar zur Gesundheitsreform: Praxisgebühr. www.die-gesund heitsreform.de/glossar/praxisgebuehr.html (in German).

Grabka, Markus M., Jonas Schreyögg, and Reinhard Busse. Die Einführung der Praxisgebühr und ihre Wirkung auf die Zahl der Arztkontakte und die Kontaktfrequenz – eine empirische Analyse. Discussion Paper 506. Berlin: German Institute for Economic Research 2005. www. diw.de/deutsch/produkte/publikationen/diskussionspapie re/docs/papers/dp50 6.pdf (abstract in English).

France: Hôpital 2007

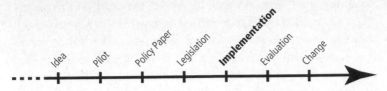

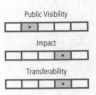

Public Visibility

Impact

Transferability

With the aim of unifying reimbursement for public and private hospitals and providing incentives for increased efficiency, France in 2004 began switching to a prospective system with "groupes homogènes de séjours," diagnosis-related groups (DRG). But a rift is threatening to develop between public and private hospitals, which had previously both supported the course adopted by the government in this matter.

To date, all public and private not-for-profit hospitals in France are financed through a global budget determined by the Ministry of Health and divided up between the regions on the basis of their populations' size, age structure and morbidity. The regional hospital agencies (Agences régionales de l'hospitalisation) then determine the individual budget of each hospital, mainly on the basis of the historical costs. Little use has so far been made of the possibility to administer a case-mix-based system.

Differences in the payments for public and private hospitals

Private for-profit hospitals, which represent 40 percent of all hospitals in France and provide about a third of the gynecological beds and half of the surgical beds, are paid according to a mixed system. This consists of a daily lump-sum payment for accommodation, care, routine medical procedures and pharmaceuticals; a separate payment for diagnostic and therapeutic procedures that depends on the level of technical equipment used; and a separate payment for blood, costly pharmaceuticals and prostheses.

Rarely has a reform in France experienced such strong support as the reorganization and harmonization of hospital reimbursement. From the point of view of the public hospitals, the previous global budget represented a rationing instrument that penalized the better-performing hospitals and did not create any space in which to react to the requirements of the public. The public hospitals had hoped that the reform would allow them considerably more autonomy.

Case mix offers advantages for all

Private hospitals, on the other hand, view the new payment structure as an opportunity to increase their share of the market. They are convinced that it will allow them to demonstrate that they can operate more cost-effectively, making them more attractive as contractual partners for the state. Measured in terms of indicators such as the number of procedures per physician or the use of operating rooms, the private hospitals are indeed already in a better position.

The French DRG system, conceived to introduce a single reimbursement system for all hospital care (with the exceptions of psychiatry and long-term care) throughout the country by 2012, represents one of the two pillars of the government's Hôpital 2007 reform plan. Hôpital 2007 is supposed to put public and private hospitals on an equal footing. But in fact, the government's hope is that increased competition will result in greater efficiency, productivity and transparency in the public sector. The second pillar of the reform, "new management," is intended to modernize the administration of public hospitals and strengthen their self-management capacity.

The initially broad support for the new reimbursement system is beginning to crumble. Both public and private hospitals complain that the government is not sticking to the time schedule it had announced and that the institutions are not being given enough leeway for their preparations. For example, payment rates for the private sector for 2005 were not published until the start of the year. Hospitals complain that there is a lack of transparency in the calculation of DRG payments, which is the responsibility of the Ministry of Health. Furthermore, they criticize the fact that the DRG payments do not take the real costs into consideration sufficiently. And finally, since it remains unclear whether the introduction of the case-mix-based payments will be accompanied by budget cuts, the hospitals are finding it difficult to assess their financial prospects.

The private and public hospitals disagree about the level of the extra budgets provided for the latter to carry out their social functions (Mission d'intérêt général et d'aide à la contractualisation, MIGAC). These include research and teaching at university clinics as well as services related to national or regional health goals (e.g., preventive care or care for special risk groups in the population). The private sector is concerned that these funds could be used to reduce deficits in the public hospitals and to provide cross-financing for medical services. For their part, the public hospitals express concern that their public duties are undervalued. As yet, no final conclusion has been reached about the level at which the ministry will set the MIGAC budget.

A final point of dispute is that the government has introduced two separate lists for payments, effectively abandoning the more daring scenario of a uniform DRG system. In the calculation of the base rate, fixed and variable costs are included for the public hospitals, but wages and medical technology services are not included for the private hospitals.

Despite all the efforts at harmonization, the payment systems for public and private hospitals in France will remain considerably different.

Sources and further reading:
Caisse nationale de l'assurance maladie des travailleurs salaires. Groupe projet tarification à l'activité. Bulletin d'informations générales N°1 2003. www.ameli.fr/dl/Infos_TAA_0403.pdf (in French).
Ministère de la Santé et des Solidarités. Plan "Hôpital 2007." www.sante.gouv.fr/htm/dossiers/hopital2007/ (in French).
Ministère de la Santé et des Solidarités. La tarification à l'activité. www.sante.gouv.fr/htm/dossiers/t2a/accueil.htm (in French).
Union Régionale des Médecin libéraux d'Ile de France. Actes colloque national T2A. 16 Juin 2004. www.urml-idf.org/urml/T2A/T2A0408.pdf (in French).

France: Ambulatory care system caught between physicians and private insurance

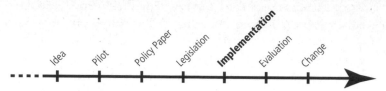

Idea   Pilot   Policy Paper   Legislation   **Implementation**   Evaluation   Change

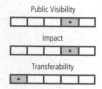

Public Visibility

Impact

Transferability

Without referral, private fees due

Two-sector agreement

In January 2005, after many years of debate, the French physicians' associations and the newly created umbrella organization of the health insurance funds (Union nationale des Caisses d'assurance maladie, UNCAM), signed a national contract on ambulatory care, opening the way for a reform of the physicians' reimbursement system and for the introduction of a gatekeeping system throughout the country. The fact that the latest health insurance reform of 2004 was linked only to certain restrictions for the medical profession allowed the physicians' associations to reach consensus with the health insurance funds.

Gatekeeping is one of the core goals of the French Health Insurance Reform Act of 2004, with which the French government wants to improve the coordination of health care services and streamline the health care system. In France, patients pay up front for all ambulatory care and then obtain a refund from their health insurance. In the past, they have been able to visit a practicing primary care physician or a specialist without any limitations. Since the reform, however, all specialists can levy private fees, which are up to 17.5 percent higher per visit or procedure if the patient has not received a referral from the practicing doctor of his or her choice (médecin traitant), who may be a general practitioner or a specialist. In other words, only those patients who are referred to a specialist by the "médecin traitant" do not have to pay private fees.

The privilege of charging patients privately is restricted to some 30 percent of the specialists and 10 percent of the general practitioners. This has repeatedly caused controversy, and not only within the medical profession. The background to this is an arrangement, in place in France since 1980, under which practicing physicians can choose between two different types of contract with the health insurance funds. Physicians in Sector 1 are entitled to charge their patients only the official fee, but in return the insurance fund pays a part of their own social insurance contributions. Physicians who choose Sector 2 do not enjoy this advantage, but they are entitled to charge additional private fees, within specific limitations.

This two-sector system seemed attractive at first, because it offered an opportunity to improve payments to physicians without burdening the public health care budget. However, objections steadily mounted that the system placed a disproportionate burden on financially disadvantaged groups in the population and gave certain physicians an advantage over others. Since the growing numbers of specialists entitled to charge private fees vehemently defended the approach, it proved difficult to control and amend.

The agreement on ambulatory care reimbursement reached in January 2005 between UNCAM and the largest association of French physicians (Confédération des syndicats médicaux français) represents more than a decisive structural alteration. The agreement also has a high symbolic value, because since 1996 all negotiations with the specialists on new reimbursement structures had failed (see issue 2 of "Health Policy Developments").

Consensus on incentive system: Breakthrough after 10 years

The result of the many years of discussions is a complicated incentive system that strengthens the position of the general practitioners but also won agreement from the specialists. Under the agreement, the "médecin traitant" receives an annual flat rate of €40 per patient for the administrative work of gatekeeping. Specialists receive a fee for the first visit that is twice the fee for a patient who has not been referred. However, if the patient visits the specialist many times within a six-month period, then no additional fee is received (apart from a small sum to cover the work involved in informing the referring physician). To motivate specialists to collaborate with the referring doctor, the system covers part of their social insurance contributions (comparable to the privilege of Sector 1 physicians). Certain services provided by eye specialists, gynecologists and psychiatrists are not affected by the gatekeeping principle.

Gatekeeping in France is thus not an obligatory mechanism—as, for example, in the Netherlands. In the various French pilot projects since the mid-1990s, only 12 percent of general practitioners and 1 percent of the population participated on a voluntary basis in physicians' networks or family doctor systems. Now, France is relying on stronger financial incentives to implement gatekeeping while maintaining the principle of free choice of physician, which is considered an important value in France.

Private insurance cover could tip the balance

Whether the "médecins traitants" will manage to establish themselves as gatekeepers will be decided above all by the private health insurance market. More than 90 percent of the population has taken out voluntary health insurance to cover the high private payments for doctors' fees, pharmaceuticals, and so forth. This could work against the core incentive of the French gatekeeping strategy. There is certainly no reason why private insurers should exclude the private fees for specialists from their insurance coverage, given that this is such an effective selling point. There is therefore considerable interest in an upcoming decree that is expected to determine whether private fees for specialist services provided without referral will be excluded by law from private insurance coverage—along the same lines as the additional co-payment of €1 introduced last year for each outpatient visit.

Sources and further reading:
Ministère des Solidarités, de la Santé et de la Famille. Réforme de l'Assurance maladie. www.assurancemaladie. sante.gouv.fr (in French).
Ministère des Solidarités, de la Santé et de la Famille. Arrêté du 3 février 2005 portant approbation de la convention nationale des médecins généralistes et des médecins spécialistes. www.medsyn.fr/mgfrance/juridique/pdf/convention2005.pdf (in French).

Patient Safety

Following the U.S. Institute of Medicine's trailblazing 1999 report *To Err Is Human,* medical error prevention and patient safety have received increasing attention and are now on the health policy agendas of many developed countries. On the basis of the first figures concerning the extent of medical errors in the United States, the Institute estimates that there are between 44,000 and 98,000 avoidable deaths among patients in hospitals each year. A series of subsequent studies from the United States, Australia and other countries shows that medical errors cause higher rates of death than traffic accidents or breast cancer and are associated with considerable costs.

Several countries have now developed strategies to optimize patient safety. Approaches in the United States focus on the testing and implementation of information technologies, on measures to identify and avoid errors, and on transparency for the public (see the reports on pages 34 and 39). Importance is attached to the strategies of Medicare and the Veterans Health Administration, which used nonpunitive reporting strategies from the aviation industry as models for health care strategies.

The Australian program, based on the recommendations of the National Advisory Group on Safety and Quality, integrates error identification and prevention in a policy of quality promotion and quality management in health care. This includes research and development on information systems across health care sectors (see the report on page 41).

Meanwhile, at the political level there is growing recognition that all the actors in the health care system need to alter their attitude to errors in medicine (see the report from Canada page 37). This means, for example, to do without the punishment of individuals as far as this is possible. It has been recognized that efforts to avoid errors in health care are particularly successful when alterations are carried out on all levels of the system.

> *Sources and further reading:*
> Institute of Medicine. *To Err Is Human: Building a Safer Health System.* Washington, D.C.: National Academy Press 1999.
> National Expert Advisory Group on Safety and Quality in Australian Health Care (NHPQ). *Implementing safety and quality enhancement in health care. National actions to support quality and safety improvement in Australian health care.* Commonwealth of Australia 1999.

United States: Patient Safety and Quality Improvement Act

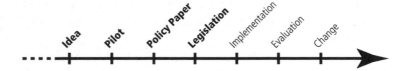

Public Visibility

Impact

Transferability

Database for patient safety

The U.S. Congress is currently debating the Patient Safety and Quality Improvement Act, searching for the right balance between the right of patients to information about medical treatment errors and the protection of individual physicians against allegations.

The act provides for physicians and other medical personnel to report medical errors or near misses to Patient Safety Organizations (PSOs) on a voluntary and anonymous basis. The reports are fed into a national patient safety database. The intention is that PSOs should analyze the data and report back on their findings to the national or regional quality improvement initiatives. The PSOs, which may be publicly or privately run, are subject to certification by the Department of Health and Human Services and are monitored by the Agency for Health Care Research and Quality.

A key component of the legislation, and the subject of controversial debate between Republicans and Democrats, is that the information submitted to the PSOs should not allow conclusions to be drawn about the person making the report, nor should it be made available for legal proceedings under civil or criminal law. Negative consequences for their career and the threat of high financial liability often keep physicians and other trained personnel from reporting medical errors, including minor complications and near misses. Experience from 21 U.S. states that have been working with error-reporting systems for several years show that inadequate reporting statistics make it considerably more difficult to introduce quality improvement policies in hospitals. **Anonymous reporting**

The origins of the Patient Safety and Quality Improvement Act lie in the recommendations of the report *To Err Is Human,* published in 1999. The data on avoidable deaths in American hospitals received considerable media coverage worldwide, and this gave rise in many countries to the inclusion of patient safety as a topic in health policies. Considerable influence was also exerted on the draft legislation by another Institute of Medicine report, *Crossing the Quality Chasm,* published in 2001. This emphasized the importance of information technology (IT) for safe, coordinated and patient-oriented care. The federal government plans to provide funding for IT-supported medical documentation and warning systems for doctors and patients. Uniform national IT standards are intended to increase safety and improve the compatibility of IT solutions, also covering electronic patient records and electronic prescriptions. **Reports of the Institute of Medicine**

The American pioneer for patient safety and IT-based quality assurance was the Veterans Health Administration (VHA). The government agency developed its successful quality program in 1997 based on the model of the NASA aviation safety reporting system. It uses computerized patient record systems (CPRS) allowing electronic communication between physicians and patients, with automated error warnings (e.g., in the case of medication interaction or necessary laboratory checks), and includes nonpunitive, anonymous reporting of complications. According to the VHA, the number of errors reported has increased 30-fold, and the system has brought a dramatic improvement in patient safety. **Pioneer: Veterans Health Administration**

The House of Representatives version of the Patient Safety Act takes the VHA experience into account and absolutely forbids the use of error reports for any purpose other than quality assurance. This means that the individual physician is protected against allegations arising from the error reports. As a result, the Republicans are guaranteed the support of representative bodies of the medical profession, such as the American Medical Association, and of the American Hospital Association.

Patient right to information

However, it seems that the last word has not yet been said. The Democrats—who traditionally see themselves as the advocate of patients' rights—worry that the law will offer loopholes for those physicians and hospitals that want to hold back on releasing information about the quality of their services, such as rates of complications and mortality. As a result, the Senate's draft of the Patient Safety Act of July 2004 allows medical error reports to be admitted in cases where the court determines they show an intention to harm.

It is now the duty of Congress to resolve the differences between the House and Senate versions. However, the greatest challenge for a national strategy for patient safety will be overcoming the practical barriers presented by the highly fragmented American health care system.

Sources and further reading:
Institute of Medicine. *Crossing the Quality Chasm: A New Health System for the 21st Century.* Washington, D.C.: National Academy Press, 2001.
Institute of Medicine. *To Err Is Human: Building a Safer Health System.* Washington, D.C.: National Academy Press, 1999.
Jha, Ashish K., Jonathan B. Perlin, Kenneth W. Kizer and R. Adams Dudley. Effect of the transformation of the Veterans Affairs health care system on the quality of care. *The New England Journal of Medicine* (348) 22 2003: 2218–2227.
National Academy for State Health Policy. How States Report Medical Errors to the Public: Issues and Barriers. www.nashp.org/_docdisp_page.cfm?LID=F5F19A94-DB2F -4C5B-B05876BE2038E891.

Canada: Institute for Patient Safety

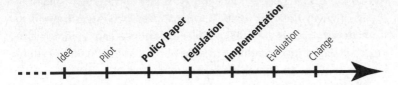

With the foundation in 2003 of the Institute for Patient Safety, Canada aims to achieve a fundamental change in attitudes to medical errors. Instead of placing the blame for critical incidents or avoidable complications on individual doctors, nurses or other personnel, the Canadian strategy places medical failures within a larger, systemic context.

Public Visibility

Impact

Transferability

On the basis of best practices from the United States, Australia and Great Britain, the Institute expects that medical personnel, in hospitals and elsewhere, would be more willing to report errors if they need not fear sanctions or negative implications for their personal career. As in the United States, computer-based, anonymous documentation systems provide assistance in reporting adverse events, medical errors or near misses. With more information, the Institute hopes to identify all the factors that coincided to cause the event (e.g., interfaces in communication and organization, levels of training, work loads and working hours of personnel) in order to eliminate weaknesses in the treatment process.

Implementing best practice

The mission of the Institute is broad and extends beyond influencing the culture of error management in medical institutions. Its duties also include analyzing existing procedures of risk management and effective intervention used in Canada and in other countries, communicating the findings to all the actors and integrating the various interested parties in activities directed towards the prevention of errors.

Focus on patient safety

The decision to place a national institute that is independent of the government in charge of safety for patients is the result of a recommendation of the National Steering Committee on Patient Safety. Founded in 2001, this committee comprised scientific experts, physicians, nurses and pharmacists, together with representatives of the government, health associations and nongovernmental organizations. It moved patient safety to the center of Canadian health policies. Previously, Baker et al. (2004) had estimated that in the year 2000, 7.5 percent of patients admitted to Canadian hospitals (185,000 people) experienced an adverse event as a consequence of medical treatment, and some 70,000 of these events could potentially have been avoided.

The 2002 National Steering Committee report entitled "Building a Safer System" laid the cornerstone for the structure and function of the Canadian Patient Safety Institute, which was founded as a not-for-profit organization in the following year. Health Canada, the Federal department for health promotion has provided C$10 million (€6.7 million) annually for patient safety initiatives which includes the work of the Institute.

It is too early to assess whether medical errors have begun to decrease in Canada following the initiatives of the Institute.

Sources and further reading:
Canadian Patient Safety Institute: www.cpsi-icsp.ca
Baker, Ross, et al. The Canadian Adverse Events Study: the incidence of adverse events among hospital patients in Canada. *Canadian Medical Association Journal* (170) 11 2004: 1678–1686.
Baker, Ross, and Peter Norton. Making Patients Safer! Reducing Error in Canadian Healthcare. *HealthCare Papers* (2) 1 2001: 10–30.
Baker, Ross, and Peter Norton. *Patient Safety and Healthcare Error in the Canadian Health Care System. A Systematic Review and Analysis of Leading Practices in Canada with Reference to Key Initiatives Elsewhere*. A Report to Health Canada. Ottawa: Health Canada, 2002.
National Steering Committee on Patient Safety. Building a Safer System: A National Integrated Strategy for Improving Patient Safety in Canadian Health Care. http://rcpsc. medical.org/publications/building_a_safer_system_e.pdf.

USA: Hospital Compare

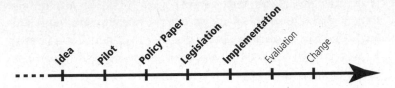

Idea — Pilot — Policy Paper — Legislation — Implementation — Evaluation — Change

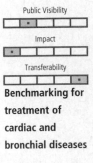

Public Visibility

Impact

Transferability

Benchmarking for treatment of cardiac and bronchial diseases

Since April 2005, the Medicare Web site Hospital Compare has been publishing data on the quality of care for patients with cardiac infarct, cardiac insufficiency and pneumonia for almost all of the 4,200 general hospitals in the United States.

Hospital Compare provides details of the extent to which each hospital follows evidence-based treatment protocols for the three diseases. The objective is to allow consumers and third-party payers to make quality comparisons of the hospitals both with each other and with the national average. The transparency is intended to motivate hospitals to ground their medical care on evidence-based recommendations and thus improve the quality of the treatment they provide. The Department of Health and Human Services plans to extend the performance measurement to the treatment of other diseases with a high prevalence and/or a high cost burden.

Public-private quality alliance

The Hospital Compare program draws primarily on a national project named "Hospital Quality Alliance: Improving Care through Information" (HQA), in which hospitals have been voluntarily publishing performance data on the Web since 2002. The key to their success is that the major hospital associations, such as the American Hospital Association and the Federation of American Hospitals, belong to this quality alliance. Physicians and consumer associations, employers and government agencies also promoted the HQA. Following the model of the HQA, Hospital Compare relies on the cooperation of public and private sectors, that is, hospital operators, physicians and consumer associations, and also the Centers for Medicare and Medicaid Services.

Business case for quality

As with many other American quality improvement policies, the roots of the Hospital Compare Initiative lie in the recommendations of the Institute of Medicine reports *To Err Is Human* and

Crossing the Quality Chasm (see report on page 34). The initiative is also fully in line with the political strategy of the Bush administration, which aims to raise awareness of health care costs and quality as part of a campaign to transfer to patients and consumers a greater financial and individual responsibility for their health (see report on page 16).

The approach arises from the assumption that competition, transparency and citizen empowerment will motivate hospitals and practicing physicians to attach greater importance to quality management. This "business case" for quality is a driving force for many other quality initiatives in the United States, such as Nursing Home Compare (a Web site for performance measurement in nursing homes) and the Health Plan Employer Data and Information Set (HEDIS®) for evaluating the quality of health plans.

Financial incentives for going public

Hospitals in the United States were very reluctant at first to make health care performance data public. Only after the Medicare Modernization Act of 2003 offered a payment premium of 0.4 percent to participating hospitals did almost all general hospitals begin to make data available to Hospital Compare. A further condition of the hospitals and physicians for supplying data was that the information should not be usable for liability litigation (see report on page 34).

More transparency—more quality?

Experts in the United States debate whether Hospital Compare's publication of performance indicators will actually improve the quality of medical treatment in hospitals. The results of studies in some states seem to support this for heart surgery or obstetrics, for example. However, the Hospital Compare site publishes mainly process data, not health outcomes, which experts regard as much more reliable and more valid quality indicators. A further disadvantage is that the Web site design and data presentation are rather complex, making it difficult for consumers to understand.

Sources and further reading:
Health Plan Employer Data and Information Set (HEDIS®): www.ncqa.org/Programs/HEDIS

Hospital Compare: www.hospitalcompare.hhs.gov/

Chassin, Marc R. Achieving and Sustaining Improved Quality: Lessons from New York State and Cardiac Surgery. *Health Affairs* (21) 4 2002: 40–51.

Hibbard, Judith H., Jean Stockard, and Martin Tusler. Does Publicizing Hospital Performance Stimulate Quality Improvement Efforts? *Health Affairs* (22) 2 2003: 84–94.

Hospital Quality Alliance. Improving Care Through Better Information. Fact Sheet. www.cms.hhs.gov/quality/hospital/HQAFactSheet.pdf.

Institute of Medicine. *Crossing the Quality Chasm: A New Health System for the 21st Century.* Washington, D.C.: National Academy Press, 2001.

Institute of Medicine. *To Err Is Human: Building a Safer Health System.* Washington, D.C.: National Academy Press, 1999.

Medicare. Nursing Home Compare. www.medicare.gov/NHCompare/Static/Related/ImportantInformation.asp?dest=NAV|Home|About|NursingHomeCompare#TabTop.

Australia: HealthConnect

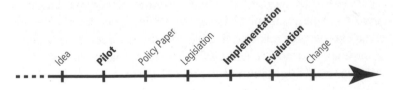

By the end of 2005, Australia aims to have developed a system of national standards for cross-sector, network-based patient records called HealthConnect. Building on a number of regional pilot projects, this program intends to meet the highest standards in terms of technology, medical content and data security.

In order to provide primary care physicians, hospitals and pharmacists with health-related information about patients rapidly and safely, five Australian states and territories (Tasmania, South Australia, Northern Territory, New South Wales and

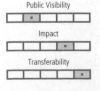

Public Visibility

Impact

Transferability

Patient records networks

41

Queensland) are currently testing models for IT networks in which health data is recorded with the consent of the patient, archived and kept available for exchange between providers. Also integrated in this system is MediConnect, a network-based documentation system for medication that is already established throughout Australia.

Report "Quality in Australian Health Care"

A keystone for the development of HealthConnect was the 1995 study "Quality in Australian Health Care," which calculated that 140,000 hospital admissions annually were the result of the inadequate application of drugs and the side effects of these pharmaceuticals. It also attributed 18,000 deaths in hospitals every year to medical errors. Australia sees the further development of information technology as one way of improving the quality and safety of medical care, because it can facilitate communication between physician and patient and between medical professionals.

National IT standards

After the pilot phase for HealthConnect, an evaluation in 2003 found the system technically feasible and practicable. The task in phase two, by the end of 2005, is to develop a national standard for the technical structure of the system so that data security can be guaranteed.

Good acceptance by patients and physicians

The project is primarily driven by politicians and IT specialists. The government's expectations that HealthConnect could increase the efficiency of health care seem to be bearing fruit. For example, South Australia has reported a decline in the number of visits to primary care physicians and the number of pathology and radiology tests ordered, which indicates that it has been possible to avoid duplication of services. In view of the high uptake rates in the study regions, it would seem that Australian physicians and patients support HealthConnect.

The long-term outcomes and the cost efficiency of HealthConnect remain unclear. Health status data are not an issue in the accompanying evaluation, which also does not determine the costs, probably high, for investing in and maintaining the new technology systems.

Sources and further reading:
HealthConnect: www.healthconnect.gov.au

Public Health

Smoking, drinking, driving too quickly, unhealthy eating, unsafe sex—these are only some of the factors that endanger the health of the population. The following chapter considers the range of public health strategies developed in various countries to meet these challenges. The second chapter then analyzes in greater depth strategies aimed at changing individual health-related behavior, such as anti-tobacco programs.

Strategies for Public Health

Public health strategies in many countries target increasing life expectancy and reducing health inequality. The specific reforms vary, however, depending on the health care system in each country and the dominant political opinions. Different countries may place different emphasis on the responsibility of the community and the individual, depending on culturally anchored views about the role of the state and the autonomy of the individual. Swedish and Finnish policies, for example, attach considerable importance to the classic health determinants such as environmental factors and social conditions. In contrast, when we consider public health programs elsewhere, the focus seems to be more on risk factors such as tobacco, alcohol and nutrition, as well as diseases such as cancer, cardiovascular disease, mental illnesses, diabetes and infections. We observe this in France (see page 45), New Zealand (see page 49), Japan (see page 53), the United States (see page 56), South Korea (see page 63) and Denmark (see page 66).

With the Public Health Act of 2004, France highlights the importance of health objectives. However, critics point out that with so many targets—one hundred in total—it will hardly be possible to implement and monitor them all effectively (see page 45).

New Zealand's strategy against cancer draws attention to the fact that the basis of every public health strategy should be to integrate all aspects of the health of the population, to implement programs across sectors and to bring together all actors in the subsequent actions (see page 49).

The example of Israel shows that prevention, health promotion and public health are becoming increasingly important in the strategic orientation of health insurance funds; it also highlights the reemergence of discussion about public versus private preventive care (see page 47).

More and more countries are trying to base political decisions on scientific evidence. In England and Wales, for example, screening programs are being tested for their effectiveness and efficiency (see page 51).

Public health interventions and their interactions with other health care policies are complex. There remains a need for closer international cooperation so that countries can learn from each other's experience.

Sources and further reading:
Allin, Sarah, Elias Mossialos, Martin McKee, and Walter Holland. *Making decisions on public health: a review of eight countries.* Brussels: European Observatory on Health Systems and Policies, 2004. Also available online at www. euro.who.int/Document/E84884.pdf.
Busse, Reinhard, and Matthias Wismar. Health target programs and health care services—any link? A conceptual and comparative study (part 1). *Health Policy* (59) 3 2002: 209–221.
Marinker, Marshall. *Health Targets in Europe: Policy, Progress and Promise.* London: BMJ Books, 2002.
Wismar, Matthias, and Reinhard Busse. Outcome-related health targets—political strategies for better health outcomes. A conceptual and comparative study (part 2). *Health Policy* (59) 3 2002: 223–241.

France: Ambitious public health policy threatened

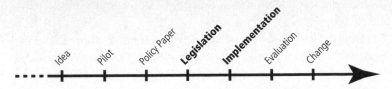

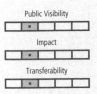

The ambitious French Public Health Act of August 2004 threatens to founder. A report from the Commission for Culture, Family and Social Affairs, commissioned by the National Assembly and published in March 2005, shows that the Act will probably not achieve the objectives within the given timeframe; the administrative implementation has already logged considerable delays within only the first six months.

New regional health alliances, ...

With the Act, France hopes to extensively reorganize its strategy for public health (see issues 1 and 3 of "Health Policy Developments"). The law defines the role of the state in public health affairs and reorganizes the responsibilities of the national and regional agencies, the numerous nongovernmental institutions and the health insurance funds. The implementation of the law will be scrutinized every year and evaluated every five years. The Act lays down health goals and specifies the processes and instruments to be used to reach these within five years. The new "Groupements regionaux de santé publique," which bring together the state administration, hospital associations and health insurance associations, are responsible for this at the regional level.

... a hundred ambitious objectives...

The annex to the Act lists a total of 100 objectives that extend over five intervention sectors: frequent diseases such as cancer and rare diseases, unhealthy behavior and environmental pollution, health inequalities, health care structures and processes (e.g., screening rates for breast cancer, antibiotics resistance, pain control), as well as health monitoring and the promotion of public health expertise.

... and bureaucracy ...

The Commission of the National Assembly blamed the level of bureaucracy for the slow progress made so far in implementation. Only 43 percent of the provisions of the law have a direct legal efficacy. The remaining 90 paragraphs (from a total of 158) will first have to be implemented in 132 decrees, ministerial orders

45

and administrative circulars. But so far the Ministry of Health administration has produced only seven documents, a fraction of those required.

Experts see themselves confirmed in their opinion that a restriction to few selected goals or a clear hierarchy of priorities would have accelerated the process. They have also criticized the fact that the law did not specify the necessary measures in each case and the financial and personnel inputs. A further difficulty has been that the Public Health Act stands in competition to the Health Insurance Reform Act passed at the same time. The minister of health is clearly treating the latter as a priority in his administration.

... threaten timely implementation

According to the Court of Accounts, drafting all the necessary texts for both laws will involve five years of legal and administrative work, so it is very doubtful whether France will be able to achieve the goals it has set itself for public health. The government must report to parliament in 2009 on the Act's impact on the general health status. However, despite the ambitious objectives of the public health strategy, the French will not be able to derive any legal rights from them.

Sources and further reading:

Assemblée nationale. Projet de loi relatif à la politique de santé publique, présenté à l'assemblé par le Ministère de la santé, de la famille et des personnes handicapées déposé le 21 mai 2003. www.assembleenationale.fr/12/projets/pl08 77.asp (in French).

Assemblée nationale. Rapport de la Commission des affaires culturelles, familiales et sociales sur la mise en application de la loi n°2004-608 du 9 août 2004 relative à la politique de santé publique. www.assembleenationale.fr/ 12/rap-info/i2207.asp (in French).

Cour des comptes. L'évolution du rôle de la Direction générale de la santé in Rapport public annuel 2004, 141–170. www.lesechos.fr/info/medias/200052615.pdf (in French).

Legifrance. Loi n°2004-806 du 9 août 2004 relative à la politique de santé publique. www.legifrance.gouv.fr/WAs pad/UnTexteDeJorf?numjo=SANX0300055L (in French).

Israel: Health plans assume responsibility for preventive care

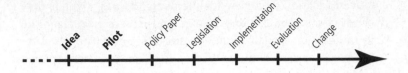

Idea · Pilot · Policy Paper · Legislation · Implementation · Evaluation · Change

In May 2005 the health plans were to assume responsibility for preventive care for all infants and schoolchildren in nine Israeli cities. This had previously been the responsibility of the public family health centers. "The original plan was modified such that the health plans will assume responsibility in three municipalities only in July 2006."

Public Visibility

Impact

Transferability

The main initiator of the reform was the Israeli Ministry of Finance, which agreed with the Ministry of Health on the pilot program as part of this year's budget legislation. In view of the economic crisis in Israel and the public health budget deficits of the Ministry of Health, one core objective is to reduce public health care expenditure. The government will no longer be providing part of the preventive care itself as in the past, but will only be financing and monitoring this.

The reform was preceded by a decade long controversy. As early as 1995, the National Health Insurance Act envisaged shifting responsibility for preventive services from the government to the health plans. The intention was to achieve greater continuity between preventive and curative care and less duplication of services, in other words, greater efficiency and effectiveness. After some health experts and consumers raised vehement objections, this provision was removed from the Act in 1998. The pilot project agreed on in March 2005 by the Knesset is a compromise, in that only a part of the preventive services previously provided by public family care centers pass over to the health plans. For the first time, the Ministry of Health will set the standards for these.

Ten-year run up to prevention pilot

However, the opponents remain undeterred in their objections to the reform. The loudest opposition comes from within the Ministry of Health itself, despite the formal support it gave to the plan. The Public Health Department argues that the current sys-

Prevention by health plans less effective?

tem is working well and thus sees no need for any changes. Opponents say the health insurance funds are oriented towards curative care and lack a view for the population as a whole; they may not be able, for example, to maintain Israel's exemplary rate of immunization against childhood diseases, now 90–92 percent.

They also argue that insufficiently or inadequately trained personnel and a shortage of equipment would make it virtually impossible for the health plans' primary care clinics to provide screening for children or individual health advice for mothers. These negative consequences would fall heavily on higher-risk groups in the population, such as people with low incomes. And, not least, civil servants in the Ministry of Health and personnel in the public family health centers are also worried about their own jobs and their occupational autonomy.

Ministry monitors quality standards

An additional annual bonus of 50 million shekels (€9 million) is intended to guarantee that the health plans provide a high level of care. To counter the reservations about quality, the funding will be contingent in part on whether the health plans meet certain targets relating, for example, to immunization rates, hearing and eye tests, house visits, maternal counseling and examinations of schoolchildren. This is the first time that the Ministry of Health has set out to monitor and regulate the services provided by the health insurance funds by setting standards.

Competitive bids for prevention contracts

The health plans are preparing for the pilot program to provide preventive care for some 14,000 infants in the three municipalities. As one effect of the reform, the plans will now be paid for some services they had previously provided at their own cost. And the plans see the reform as an opportunity to attract families with children, a preferred group of customers.

In view of the lengthy political process and the ongoing debate, the Ministry of Finance agreed with the Ministry of Health that there should be a comprehensive evaluation of the pilot project.

The Myers-JDC-Brookdale Institute has already produced a draft for the study, covering the measurement of structure, processes and outcome indicators. A study by Palti et al. (2004) found no significant differences in the quality of care or in the satisfaction of mothers. This suggests that mother and child preventive care provided by the health plans is at least comparable with that provided by the public family health centers.

48

Sources and further reading:
Ministry of Finance. Pilot Plan for Transferring Responsibility for Family Health Centers and Preventive Care in Schools to the Health Plans. Jerusalem, February 2005 (in Hebrew).
Palti, Hava, Rosa Gofin, and Bella Adler. Evaluation of use of family health centers: personal and systemic factors. *Harefu'a* (134) 32004: 184–188 (in Hebrew).
Rosen, Bruce. Proposal for an Evaluation of the Pilot Program in the Public Health Care Services. Jerusalem: Myers-JDC-Brookdale Institute, 2005 (in Hebrew).

New Zealand: Cancer control action plan

In March 2005, the New Zealand Ministry of Health presented a detailed action plan with the goal of controlling cancer. Cancer diseases, and in particular carcinoma of the lung, breast, bowel, and prostate gland, are responsible for some 30 percent of all deaths in New Zealand, having overtaken cardiovascular diseases as the leading cause of death.

In 2003, the government defined a Cancer Control Strategy that outlined six goals: preventing lifestyle-related, infectious and work-related health risks; ensuring effective screening programs; ensuring effective diagnosis and treatment; improving quality of life for cancer patients and their families by social support, rehabilitation and palliative care; improving the delivery of services across the continuum of cancer care; and improving the effectiveness of cancer control through research and surveillance.

Anticancer strategy: From prevention to palliative medicine

The ministry appointed a working group, made up of prevention experts, clinical specialists and also of consumers and patient groups, that developed a plan outlining an impressive array of actions. For all sectors, the Action Plan 2005–2010 determined secondary goals, defined target outcomes, specified steps for actions by the actors and the interest groups and established milestones across the next five-year period.

In the style of the governing Labour-led coalition, which since 1999 has targeted its health policies to specific populations, the cancer control action plan pays special attention to ethnic minorities. Ethnicity, socioeconomic status, gender and place of residence are the most important determinants for the health status and life expectancy of a New Zealander. Various factors contribute to health inequalities, among them the patient's knowledge, outlook on life and financial background, and at the systemic level, access to and quality of medical services. In 2000, the age-adjusted mortality rate for cancer among Maori men was 51 percent higher than among other New Zealanders, and for Maori women it was 82 percent higher. As one of its objectives, the government intends to increase the screening rate for breast cancer of Maori women 55 to 74 years old from 45 to 70 percent.

A further key goal of the New Zealand cancer control strategy is to achieve a continuum of cancer control across the entire healthcare spectrum. From prevention through to palliative medicine, the action plan ties in many public and nongovernmental organizations. Through an integrated approach to the planning, development and provision of measures, the plan aims to reduce gaps in the care provided, as well as to reduce overlaps in service. The first step is to establish tumor networks throughout the country, which the government views as a way to coordinate services better and make more efficient use of scarce resources.

According to experts, the key problems of the cancer control plan lie not in its strategic orientation, which enjoys broad support in New Zealand, but in its complexity and its many different individual aspects. The success of New Zealand's strategy will depend above all on whether the newly established Cancer Control Council manages to bring together the numerous stakeholders—government agencies and administration, patients and families, planners, funders and service providers—across sectoral boundaries and to coordinate them in controlling cancer.

Sources and further reading:
Ministry of Health. The Cancer Control Action Plan. www.moh.govt.nz/moh.nsf/49ba80c00757b8804c2566730 01d47d0/abed0ba681a637e1cc256fbc006f22d7?OpenDocument.
Ministry of Health. The Cancer Control Strategy.

England: National screening program for bowel cancer

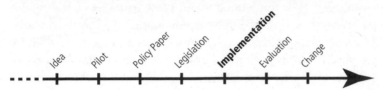

In April 2006, England will launch a national screening program for bowel cancer. For the first time, men and women will be entitled to regular screening for occult blood in feces. A sigmoidoscopy (endoscopic inspection of the lower third of the large intestine) every 10 years is the second component of the scheme for early detection of colorectal tumors. Since policies against cancer in Great Britain are widely supported, no resistance to the screening program for bowel cancer is anticipated.

As in New Zealand, the government had already formulated a National Cancer Plan in 2000, specifying targets and standards for prevention, medical care and palliative medicine for the most frequent types of cancer. The government is now implementing population-related screening for bowel cancer, which has proved to be successful in pilot studies. In Great Britain, endoscopic screening for colorectal cancer is currently proposed once every ten years for people above 60 years of age. The reports on the final evaluation of the effectiveness of the sigmoidoscopy for 50-year olds have not yet been completed.

Colorectal cancer is the third most common form of cancer for men in Great Britain, after prostate and lung cancer, and the second most common form for women, after breast cancer. An early diagnosis of bowel cancer or self-diagnosis is difficult be-

Public Visibility

Impact

Transferability

Endoscopy from 60 years of age

Bowel cancer mortality high in European comparison

cause of the long period with no clear symptoms and the unspecific course of disease. Despite a general downward trend in the mortality attributed to malignant neoplasms, the United Kingdom has a high mortality rate from bowel cancer in comparison with other European countries. Furthermore, the tumors are diagnosed at a relatively late stage.

Unnecessarily delayed diagnosis

One reason for the delay in diagnosis in Great Britain is a shortage of qualified endoscopists, which means long waiting times for endoscopic examinations and the widespread use of less sensitive radiological methods.

In order to do something about these bottlenecks, the British government is investing the largest part of the colorectal carcinoma screening budget of €55 million in a program of training for physicians. By the end of 2005, at least 345 additional endoscopists are to be trained in seven regional and three national centers.

It remains to be seen whether the new screening program can reduce the bowel cancer mortality rate in Great Britain by 15 percentage points, as the reports of the pilot programs predicted.

Sources and further reading:
Department of Health. National Service Frameworks. www.dh.gov.uk/PolicyAndGuidance/HealthAndSocialCare Topics/HealthAndSocialCareArticle/fs/en?CONTENT_ID= 4070951&chk=W3ar/W
Department of Health. The NHS Cancer Plan. www.dh. gov. uk/ Publications And Statistics/ Publications/ Publica tionsPolicyAndGuidance/PublicationsPolicyAndGuidance Article/fs/en?CONTENT_ID=4009609&chk=n4LXTU.
Department of Health. The NHS Plan. www.dh.gov.uk/ PolicyAndGuidance/OrganisationPolicy/Modernisation/N HSPlan/fs/en?CONTENT_ID=4082690 &chk=/DU1UD.
Department of Health. Reid announces new national screening programme to tackle bowel cancer. Press release 27 October 2004. www.dh.gov.uk/PublicationsAndStatis tics/PressReleases/PressReleasesNotices/fs/en?CONTENT _ID=4092376&chk=F1jw5w.

Japan: Ban on blood donations against new variant Creutzfeldt-Jakob disease

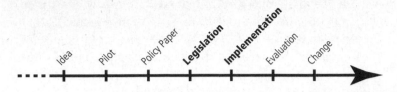

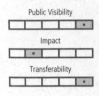

In reaction to the death of the first Japanese man of new variant Creutzfeldt-Jakob disease (vCJD), Japan introduced a strict ban on blood donations from people who had spent time in European countries in May 2005. The Japanese man who died in December 2004 from the transmissible spongiform encephalopathy may possibly have contracted this from BSE-contaminated meat in 1990 during a stay of several days in Great Britain and France.

The variant CJD was first described in 1996 in England. In contrast to the conventional form of Creutzfeldt-Jakob disease, the variant affects young people in particular. As of April 2005, a total of 149 people had died of vCJD in Great Britain and nine people in France. Individual cases of vCJD have also been reported in Canada, Ireland, Italy and the United States.

Experiments with animals suggest the possibility that the infectious agent—an atypical protein (prion) that also causes BSE (bovine spongiform encephalopathy)—could be transmitted by blood transfusions. There is no confirmed or suspected case to date of vCJD transmission by means of blood or blood products. As a precautionary measure, however, in 2001 Germany and Great Britain began requiring that white blood cells be filtered out of the blood prior to transfusion (leukocyte depletion). Since there are concerns that even cell-free plasma could transmit the disease, Australia, Canada, Switzerland and the United States have banned blood donations from people who have spent time in countries with a high BSE risk.

Although public interest in BSE and vCJD has declined markedly in Europe, the first death in Japan received considerable national media coverage there, so that the Ministry of Health, Work and Welfare came under great pressure to act.

Media coverage obliges government to act

In May 2005, the Ministry announced a strict ban on blood

Risk-related ban
on blood dona-
tions ...

donations by people who had spent more than one day in Great Britain or France between 1980 and 1996. It is estimated that this will exclude that 2 to 6 percent of donors. However, restrictions also apply to other countries in the European region. In all, 36 countries were assigned to five categories that vary in the length of stay allowed before blood donation is banned. For example, anybody who spent more than half a year in the period 1980–2004 in Germany, Ireland, Italy, the Netherlands, Spain, Belgium or Portugal cannot donate blood in Japan now.

... leads to acute
shortage of blood
products

As medical experts from the Red Cross and the hospitals feared, this has already led to a worrisome shortage of blood products in Japan. It is questionable whether the April 2005 appeal from the Ministry of Health to donate more blood will suffice to restock the reserves, which have shrunk to 80 percent of the average national three-day supply. The ministry has therefore announced that it may relax the ban on donations from travelers who had spent time in low-risk countries.

Sources and further reading:
WHO. Variant Creutzfeldt-Jakob Disease. Factsheet N° 180.
www.who.int/mediacentre/factsheets/fs180/en/index.html.

Healthy Lifestyles

Obesity, according to the WHO, is one of the most underestimated and neglected health risks worldwide.

In the United States, which has 60 million obese inhabitants, obesity has reached epidemic proportions. California Governor Arnold Schwarzenegger has launched an initiative against excessive overweight, pointing to the state's highly successful anti-tobacco campaign (see page 56). Funds from the tobacco tax were carefully targeted to effective programs, with strict implementation and coordination under state guidance. Over the past twenty years, the campaign transformed the social attitudes to smoking and the framework conditions in California to such an extent that in 2003 only 16.2 percent of the state population smoked, almost 10 percentage points less than in 1984.

In Europe, the rate of smokers dropped from 45 to 30 percent in the past 30 years. In contrast, the prevalence of smoking in eastern European countries, and particularly in the Baltic States, has continued to increase steadily among young people and women. According to the 2002 World Health Organization Report "Reducing Risks, Promoting Healthy Life," tobacco use still remains the leading avoidable cause of death in the industrialized nations.

International experience shows that price increases and tax hikes are the most effective instruments to reduce the consumption of legal addictive substances. But fiscal approaches to tobacco control regularly come into conflict with the economic interests of businesses and the government in promoting employment, economic growth and tax revenue. In one of the negative effects of EU expansion, Finland finds itself obliged to reduce the tax on alcohol by 30 percent, removing one of the main pillars of the Scandinavian strategy against alcohol-related illness, accidents and acts of violence (see page 59). In South Korea, the government stands accused of failing to act in accordance with its statement of intent and shift the extra revenues from the tobacco tax to support anti-tobacco initiatives (see page 63).

Most effective: price increases

Scientists agree on the health risks posed by passive smoking. An increasing number of countries, such as Ireland, Italy, Malta, New Zealand, Norway, Singapore and Sweden, have therefore introduced a complete ban on smoking in public and at work. Similar regulations have been announced in other countries, among them Australia, Czech Republic, England, Finland, Hungary, Portugal, Scotland and Spain. The bans on smoking have been implemented with varying degrees of success against opposition and vested interests, including the hospitality industry (see reports from Spain, New Zealand and Denmark, pages 61, 64 and 66).

Sources and further reading:
WHO. Framework Convention on Tobacco Control. www.who.int/tobacco/fctc/text/final/en/.
WHO. The World Health Report 2002—Reducing Risks, Promoting Healthy Life. www.who.int/whr/2002/en/index.html.

WHO Regional Office for Europe. Tobacco Control Database. http://data.euro.who.int/tobacco/?TabID=2402.
WHO Regional Office for Europe. Tobacco-free Europe. www.euro.who.int/eprise/main/who/progs/tob.

California: Obesity Prevention Initiative

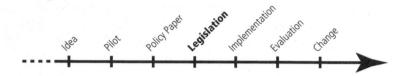

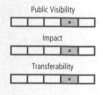

Public Visibility

Impact

Transferability

Schwarzenegger's strategy: healthy eating and exercise

Obesity: Alarming figures

Governor Arnold Schwarzenegger wants California to play a leading role in turning round the rapid increase in obesity in the population. To establish the Department of Health Services (DHS) as the central coordinator and financing agency for obesity prevention and treatment, Schwarzenegger announced an investment of $6 million (€5 million) in April 2005.

Possibly influenced by his own philosophy of physical fitness, Schwarzenegger's strategy focuses on two core goals: healthy nutrition and exercise. More than half the budget of the California Obesity Initiative is earmarked for suitable community-based projects. The plan calls for putting $1.4 million (€1.2 million) into anti-obesity programs of Medi-Cal, the Californian state health plan for the poor. Much smaller sums of $150,000 (€124,000) each will be spent on education campaigns and promoting health at work. Finally, half a million dollars (€413,000) is earmarked for public research projects to analyze epidemiological trends, evaluate the effect of the program interventions and identify future policy options and solutions.

The California Obesity Initiative comes in response to the dramatic extent of the "obesity epidemic" in the United States. The latest figures from the National Center for Health Statistics show that 30 percent of Americans above the age of 20 years, more than 60 million adults, are obese.

In comparison with other states, this trend towards overweight is most pronounced in California. More than half the adults and about a quarter of children there are obese. Associated and secondary illnesses such as diabetes mellitus, arterial hypertension and cardiovascular disease are on the rise.

Obesity is not only a serious public health problem in California; it is also costly. A study commissioned by the California DHS and published in April 2005, "The Economic Costs of Physical Inactivity, Obesity and Overweight in Californian Adults," which received wide media coverage at the time, calculated health costs and lost productivity amounting to $22 billion (€18 billion) per annum for the state and predicted that in 2005 the toll would rise to $28 billion (€23 billion).

Excess weight is costly

The U.S. Centers for Disease Control and Prevention (CDC) had set the goal in 2000 of reducing the prevalence of obesity over the next decade to below 15 percent. Under its Nutrition and Physical Activity Program to Prevent Obesity and Other Chronic Diseases, the CDC currently cofinances prevention initiatives in 28 federal states.

Fight against obesity is a national health objective

The U.S. Department of Health and Human Services has recognized obesity as an illness. Since July 2004, Medicare has provided coverage for treatment of obesity.

The campaign against obesity in California has been characterized by a number of individual and usually uncoordinated efforts. The dedication of volunteers led to the emergence of a wide range of community-based organizations, primarily funded by federal subsidies or private donations. For example, California Endowment, a private foundation, promised $26 million (€22 million) in March 2005 for programs to counter obesity in children.

Partial solutions in California

The California authorities have been active in the past with isolated measures that have tended to be under-funded (see "Ban on soft drinks at schools" in issue 3 of "Health Policy Developments"). The most important exception is the project "Leaders Encouraging Activity and Nutrition" (LEAN), in which the DHS and the not-for-profit Public Health Institute coordinated community activities. LEAN led the planning commission established in 2000 to develop a Californian strategy against obesity (California Obesity Prevention Initiative), and their action plan formed part of the basis for Schwarzenegger's current initiative.

As the California senate debates the budget plans for 2005–

2006, Schwarzenegger must defend his initiative in a tight budget situation. Some senators question the level of the proposed anti-obesity budget and also criticize the state's leading role in the organization.

Model: anti-
tobacco campaign

The governor and supporters of the proposals, such as representatives of the medical profession, draw attention to the highly successful precedent of the California anti-tobacco campaign. Since 1988, the state has raised money through a cigarette tax and used the earmarked funds to run a comprehensive, multi-agency tobacco reduction program. As a result, the proportion of smokers in California fell from 25.8 percent in 1984 to 16.2 percent in 2003.

To repeat this Californian success story, the campaign against obesity must also manage to raise public awareness, stimulate a review of social standards and individual behavior and bring about a sustainable transformation of living and working conditions, in accordance with the motto "Make the healthier choice the easier choice."

Sources and further reading:
California Obesity Initiative: http://govbud.dof.ca.gov/ Budget Summary/ MAJOR PROGRAM AREAS/ Healthand HumanServices/section2 _4.html
California Obesity Prevention Initiative: www.dhs.ca.gov/ ps/cdic/copi/default.htm
Centers for Disease Control and Prevention, Nutrition and Physical Activity Division: www.cdc.gov/nccdphp/dnpa/ obesity
Leaders Encouraging Activity and Nutrition (LEAN): www.californiaprojectlean.org
Chenoweth, David. The Economic Costs of Physical Inactivity, Obesity, and Overweight in California Adults: Health Care, Workers Compensation, and Lost Productivity. Study for the California Department of Health Services, 2005. www.dhs. ca. gov/ ps/ cdic/ cpns/ press/ downloads/ Cost of ObesityToplineReport.pdf.

Finland: Major reduction in alcohol tax

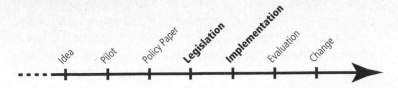

Idea   Pilot   Policy Paper   **Legislation**   **Implementation**   Evaluation   Change

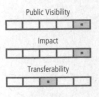

Public Visibility

Impact

Transferability

Finland abandoned its traditionally restrictive alcohol policies in March 2004 and introduced extensive cuts in the taxes on alcoholic beverages. With the program Alcohol Prevention 2004–2007, the Finnish Ministry for Social Affairs and Health is now counteracting the expected jump in alcohol consumption.

EU regulation: increasing alcohol consumption

The Finnish Ministry of Finance found itself obliged to reduce the duties on spirits, wines and beer by 44 percent, 32 percent and 10 percent, respectively, because the common market regulations within the European Union made it impossible to restrict the amount of privately imported alcohol.

After a ten percent reduction in alcohol consumption in the early 1990s, the Finns were back at an average equivalent total consumption of almost 9 liters of pure ethanol by 1995, the peak level of national consumption in 1990. Deaths due to alcohol-associated illness and poisoning continue to rise steadily.

Exacerbated alcohol problem as Estonia joins EU

The liberalization of imports from the Baltic States has further exacerbated this trend. Estonia is only a two-hour ferry trip from Helsinki, and since Estonia joined the European Union in May 2004, Finns have been able to legally import unlimited quantities of alcoholic drinks for private consumption at prices as much as 50 percent below the prices in Finland.

Since the importation of alcohol from EU member states cannot be banned or otherwise discriminated against by duties or other measures, Finland had to lift its strict import limitations of one liter of spirits and five liters of wine in January 2004. Like its neighbor Sweden, Finland had been granted transitional agreements in its own EU accession negotiations in 1995, but these expired at the end of 2003. Since then, Finns have been able to import from other EU member states up to 110 liters of beer, 90 liters of wine, 10 liters of spirits and 20 liters of other alcoholic beverages without import duties. Moreover, these amounts are

59

interpreted by Finnish authorities to be only indicative limits rather than real ones.

In the government's view, the massive reduction in domestic alcohol prices was the best of the bad options available. Unless it took steps to ensure that most alcoholic beverages continued to be purchased in Finland, it would lose too much revenue from the value-added tax. Objections by health policy experts were crowded out as the debate concentrated on tax losses, the falling retail sales of the distilling and brewing industries and the threat of job losses.

Battling temptation with a prevention program

Since the tax cuts in March 2004, prices for spirits have fallen by 36 percent, and for wine and beer by 13 percent and 3 percent, respectively. The Ministry for Social Affairs and Health estimates that alcohol consumption will increase by 15 percent. With the alcohol prevention program published in April 2004, the ministry aims to turn this trend around. In order to prevent rises in alcohol-related illness, accidents and violence, various organizations and actors are to enter into voluntary formal partnership agreements and undertake to focus in particular on alcohol prevention for children and in the family.

The ministry hopes that the coordination and combination of programs in local communities, enterprises, businesses, the church and nongovernmental organizations will prove more effective than other measures in the past. And one pillar of the Finnish alcohol policy has remained unaffected. The state alcohol monopolist Alko, with its 320 outlets throughout the country, still retains exclusive rights to the retail sale of all products with an alcohol content of more than 4.7 percent. At the start of 2006, the Ministry of Health will present parliament with the first results of the alcohol program and an assessment of its success. It will then become clear whether Finland is able to counteract the severe impact on its health policies of its accession to the European Union.

Sources and further reading:
Ministry of Social Affairs and Health. Alcohol Programme 2004–2007. www. stm. fi / Resource. phx / eng / strag / progr / alcohol/alcohol.htx (in Finnish and Swedish, summary in English).

Spain: Anti-tobacco law

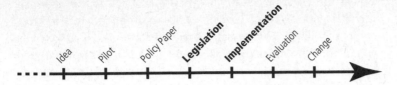

The Spanish parliament is about to pass a national anti-tobacco law that will come into force at the beginning of 2006. Recent tax increases on tobacco have taken place, and the Government is considering even more tax rises due to the reduction of prices just implemented by foreign tobacco firms (January 2006). However, in the opinion of health experts, the bundle of reforms is not really suited to bring about any significant reduction in tobacco-related illnesses and their costs in Spain.

The bill presented by the Socialist government under José Luis Zapatero introduces a nationwide ban on the sale or distribution of tobacco products to young people below the age of 18 years. This would harmonize the regulations in the different regions of Spain. At the same time, the law would implement at the national level the requirements of the EU directive banning tobacco advertising on the radio and television, in the press, via the Internet and by sponsorships.

The third basic element of the law is the ban on smoking at work and in restaurants, bars and hotels. Hotel managers and restaurant owners fear that this restriction will keep guests away. As a concession, the law applies only to buildings and premises with more than 100 square meters of floor space. As a result, guests and employees in most of Spain's bars and bistros are still exposed to second-hand smoke, since there is no requirement to provide a smoke-free area. The government did not accept the argument that in other countries a general ban on smoking has by no means had a negative impact on sales and numbers of guests.

Ban on smoking ineffective due to special provisions

In a European comparison, Spanish tobacco prices are extremely low. A further weakness of the Spanish initiative is that the reform package no longer includes an increase in the tax on tobacco. Although the current bill corresponds to the draft

No increase in tobacco tax

Public Visibility

Impact

Transferability

proposed by the previous government under Aznar's Partido Popular in January 2003, the tax increase, which is the responsibility of the Ministry of Finance, has been dropped. Health policy experts see this as a concession to the tobacco industry and to the Ministry of Economics and Labor, which had successfully argued that there could be risks of a black market and tobacco smuggling, lower sales, job losses and rising inflation.

Regional variations in implementation

In the final analysis, the impact of the Act will depend on how it is implemented at the local level, because public health concerns in Spain are the financial and organizational responsibility of the regions. Some local governments have already developed reporting systems for citizens and are planning systems of fines to penalize breaches of the smoking ban. The central government has recently announced that it will make an additional €37 million available to the regions for preventive health care policies, which also include the anti-tobacco measures. Despite their autonomy, the regions still have to provide the central government with accounts of how they have used the resources.

The proposed law is without doubt a first step towards facing up to the tobacco problem in Spain. However, from the point of view of many public health experts and medical specialists, the initiative is too weak and not ambitious enough, because it stops short of a general ban on smoking, does not increase the tobacco tax, and makes no provisions for campaigns, programs to promote giving up smoking or courses for training personnel.

Sources and further reading:
Ministerio de Sanidad y Consumo. Plan Nacional de Prevención y Control del Tabaquismo 2003–2007. Madrid 2003 (in Spanish).
Villalbí, Joan. Políticas para reducir el daño que causa el tabaco. *Adicciones* 16, Suppl. 2, 2004: 379–390 (in Spanish).

South Korea: Tobacco tax and health promotion

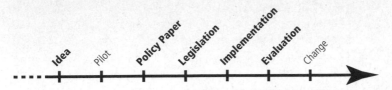

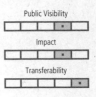

Public Visibility

Impact

Transferability

The January 2005 increase in the tobacco tax in South Korea had the desired effect, as the first figures on smoking behavior show. According to a survey, almost 1 percent of the male population gave up smoking in the first three months after the tax increase.

Although these results cannot provide a firm basis for predicting any long-term effects, the Ministry of Health and Welfare still feels confirmed in its tobacco prevention strategy.

However, the health minister's proposal to raise the tobacco tax again this year has so far been successfully opposed by the Ministry of Finance and Economy. In December 2004, after a lengthy dispute, the two ministries had reached an agreement (see issue 3 of "Health Policy Developments") that meant an increase of €0.40 per pack. This was only about a quarter of the increase originally proposed by the health minister, who had sought to more than double the cost of a pack of cigarettes.

Conflict between prevention and state revenues continues

The bitter resistance from the Ministry of Finance is based on the fear that if the numbers of smokers fell, the authorities would face a considerable loss of income.

Revenue earmarked ...

Ten percent of the tobacco tax is earmarked for the state Health Promotion Fund and therefore not readily available for the public coffers.

There is currently considerable debate about how the money in the fund is utilized. The national health insurance system is in a financial crisis, with no sign at the moment of increases in contributions. A large proportion of the money in the Health Promotion Fund is therefore being tapped to close the gaps in the budgets of the health insurance funds, although these have a primarily curative orientation. Critics argue that with this cross-financing, the Fund is going counter to its original purpose, while projects and institutions involved in health promotion are not receiving adequate support.

... but still diverted elsewhere

Sources and further reading:
Ministry of Health and Welfare: http://english.mohw.go.
kr/index.jsp

New Zealand: 100 percent smoke-free

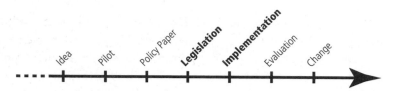

Public Visibility

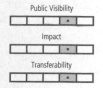

Impact

Transferability

100-percent ban on smoking

As the fifth country worldwide, New Zealand introduced an absolute ban on smoking in public on December 10, 2004.

Second-hand smoke has been completely banned from bars, restaurants, cafes, clubs and casinos, department stores, public transport and taxis, offices, factories and workplaces. Within a one-year transitional period, all designated smoking areas in buildings must be closed or moved outside. The only exceptions to the strict ban on smoking are rooms with a private, "domestic" character in hotels, care homes for the elderly, hospitals and prisons.

Growing acceptance in hospitality industry

Despite the mounting evidence showing the health impact of second-hand smoke, the New Zealand government managed to enforce a ban on smoking in public places only after a number of years of controversial debate. The most vociferous opponents were from bars, restaurants, hotels, and the entertainment industry. In particular, bar and club owners were worried that they would lose guests and their sales would fall. According to a survey, however, 57 percent of bar owners accepted the right of their employees to a smoke-free working environment, and only a quarter of managers expected negative long-term financial consequences.

Smoking: Health risk number one

The proportion of New Zealanders who smoke has fallen from 30 percent at the end of the 1980s to some 25 percent now. However, the figure for young people is 26 percent, 33 percent for people with low income and 49 percent for members of the Maori ethnic group. Thus, tobacco can still contribute significantly to the poorer health status of specific groups of the population.

With the strict implementation of the policy protecting nonsmokers, New Zealand is continuing the course it began in 1990 with the Smoke-free Environment Act, which exiled smokers at work to separate rooms. Since then, New Zealand has banned the sale of tobacco to minors and placed restrictions on advertising and the promotion of cigarettes. Tobacco companies were obliged to declare the composition of their products and the additives they contain.

A 15-year tradition of protecting nonsmokers

In the New Zealand Health Strategy of 2000, New Zealand declared the continued campaign against tobacco as one of 13 objectives for the health system. The five-year program "Clearing the Smoke" aims to follow the ban on smoking by 2009 with higher tobacco taxes, an extension of the ban on advertising and marketing, stricter implementation of the ban on sales to minors under 18, a reduction in the nicotine content in cigarettes, increased promotion of health in schools, and by campaigns in the mass media.

"Clearing the Smoke"

The government intends to monitor successes and negative effects of the ban on smoking. Indicators will be trends in the sales figures for tobacco and alcohol (considered an alternative drug), as well as the impact of the ban on tourism and employment figures. An initial assessment announced for the start of 2006 will show the extent to which the ban on smoking is being followed and how it is viewed in opinion polls. Health examinations, such as measurement of urine levels of cotinine (a metabolic product of nicotine), would indicate whether the smoking habits of New Zealanders have changed. Experts think it probable that smoke-free could soon become the standard in New Zealand.

Sources and further reading:
National Drug Policy: www.ndp.govt.nz
Ministry of Health. Clearing the Smoke: A five-year plan for tobacco control in New Zealand. Wellington 2004. www.moh.govt.nz/moh.nsf/49ba80c00757b8804c2566730 01d47d0/aafc588b348744b9cc256f39006eb29e?OpenDoc ument.

Ministry of Health. The New Zealand National Health Strategy 2000. www.moh.govt.nz/moh.nsf/ea6005dc347e 7bd44c2566a40079ae6f/fb62475d5d911e88cc256d42007bd6 7e?OpenDocument.
Ministry of Health. Smokefree Law in New Zealand. www.moh.govt.nz/smokefreelaw.

Denmark: More signs instead of less smoke

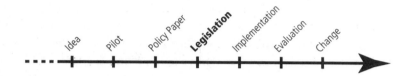

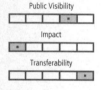

Far from imposing a complete ban on smoking, as New Zealand did, the Danish government is relying on the power of the people to implement effective protection for nonsmokers. According to a draft bill proposed by the right-liberal government in November 2004, restaurants and bars face fines if they do not have a sign stating whether their premises are totally, partially, or not smoke-free. Previously they only had to provide this information to guests on demand.

Competition creates non-smoker protection ...
According to the government's classic-liberal ideas, the Danes will use their power as informed customers and employees to decide in favor of smoke-free establishments. They will thus exert sufficient market pressure on other establishments to adopt measures to protect nonsmokers. However, public health experts consider it unlikely that the Danish approach will prove very effective, because the newly introduced signs will not persuade many Danes to switch restaurants or to visit another bar. Restaurants with smoke-free areas are already using this as a marketing strategy.

... or no change?
The proposed legislation can be implemented relatively easily, and the political opposition also regards it as an appropriate starting point for raising public awareness about passive smoking. However, the Social Democrats emphasize that in the event

66

of a change of government, they will endeavor to implement a smoking ban like that in other countries. Since the Danes reelected the government in early elections in February 2005, however, a change of course in health policies seems unlikely at present.

Sources and further reading:
Ministry of the Interior and Health. Forslag til lov om ændring af lov om røgfri miljøer i offentlige lokaler, transportmidler og lignende. www.im.dk/Index/dokumenter. asp?o=85&n=1&h=19&t=1&d=2394&s=4 (in Danish).

Pharmaceutical policy and drug evaluation

In many developed countries, expenditure on pharmaceuticals is growing disproportionately in comparison with expenditures on other health sectors such as outpatient or hospital care. In this context, one bone of contention is the "me too" products, new drugs that offer no or only marginal additional benefits compared to pharmaceuticals already on the market.

Many countries have therefore introduced a post-licensing evaluation before making decisions on a drug's price, eligibility for reimbursement and recommendation of its use in clinical guidelines. The number of public institutions or evaluation committees assessing evidence for the added value of a drug in comparison to other available therapies has grown continuously over the past decade (see table below).

National drug review bodies and expert committees

Country	Drug review body, expert commitee	Comparative evaluation of pharmaceuticals since
Australia	Pharmaceutical Benefits Advisory Committee, Economic Sub-committee	1987
Canada (pricing)	Patented Medicine Prices Review Board, PMPRB's Human and Veterinary Drug Advisory Panels	1994

Switzerland	Swiss Federal Office of Public Health, Confederate Pharmaceutivcal Commission (Bundesamt für Gesundheit, Eidgenössische Arzneimittelkommission)	1994
Netherlands	Health Care Insurance Board, Commitee for Pharmaceutical Aid (College voor zorgverzekeringen, Commissie Farmaceutische Hulp)	1996
United Kingdom (England and Wales)	National Institute for Clinical Excellence	1999
Finland	Pharmaceuticals Pricing Board (Lääkkeiden hintalautakunta)	1999
France	Comité économique des produits de santé, Commission de Transparence	1999
New Zealand	Pharmaceutical Management Agency, Pharmacology and Therapeutic Advisory Committee	2000
Norway	Norwegian Medicines Agency (Statens Legemiddelverk), Department of Pharmacoeconomics	2002
Sweden	Pharmaceutical Benefits Board (Läkemedelsförmånsnämnden), PBB-Committee, PBB-projectgroup	2002
Canada (reimbursement)	Canadian Expert Drug Advisory Committee, Common Drug Review Directorate at the Canadian Coordinating Office for Health Technology Assessment	2003
Austria	Federation of Austrian Social Security Institutions, Pharmaceutical Evaluation Committee (Hauptverband der Österreichischen Sozialversicherungsträger, Heilmittel-Evaluierungs-Kommission)	2003
Germany	Institute for Quality and Efficiency in Health Care (Institut für Qualität und Wirtschaftlichkeit im Gesundheitswesen)	2004

Source: Zentner, Velasco-Garrido and Busse 2005

Following the example set by Australia in 1993, there is a worldwide trend to establish not only effectiveness but also cost-effectiveness as an evaluation criterion (see report on Denmark in issue 2 of "Health Policy Developments"). In this context, the report from Finland (see page 76) shows the problems that can be caused by a costly drug therapy whose beneficial long-term effects are dubious. In accordance with the so-called "rule of rescue," society is often prepared to spend a lot of money on an individual whose life is in danger or for whom treatment would not previously have been possible.

Developed countries, however, face the challenge of having to clarify not only whether a new drug should be regarded as a therapeutic improvement, but also how those innovations can be rewarded and incentives provided for manufacturers to invest in research and development. Instruments increasingly used include listing a pharmaceutical on positive lists or preferred drugs lists (see reports from the United States and Spain, pages 74 and 78) and agreeing on higher drug prices.

Negative decisions are always a cause for the pharmaceutical industry to criticize the lengthy evaluation procedures and the quality of the evidence-based evaluations. It is not uncommon for decisions to be contested successfully in litigation (see report on France in issue 2 of "Health Policy Developments"). The example of Australia (see page 71) demonstrates how public drug evaluation and regulation increasingly come into conflict with a global market. The free trade agreement with the United States obliges Australia to allow an independent assessor to review negative decisions by its state Pharmaceutical Benefits Advisory Committee.

One of the challenges facing pharmaceutical policy-makers is therefore the need to develop international standards and uniform methods of evidence-based drug evaluation and to increase the transparency of the procedures and policy decisions.

Sources and further reading:
Mossialos, Elias, Monique Mrazek, and Tom Walley (eds.). *Regulating pharmaceuticals in Europe: striving for efficiency, equity and quality.* Berkshire: Open University Press, 2004.

Also available online at www.euro.who.int/document/
E83015.pdf.
Zentner, Annette, Marcial Velasco-Garrido, and Reinhard
Busse. *Methoden der vergleichenden Bewertung pharmazeuti-
scher Produkte.* www.egms.de/en/journals/hta/2005-1/hta
000009.shtml (abstract and executive summary in English).

Australia: Drug evaluation and free trade agreement with the USA

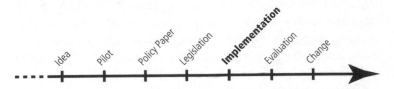

As a result of the free trade agreement signed in May 2004 with the United States, Australia has reformed part of its drug evaluation process by which it decides whether consumer costs for a new pharmaceutical will be publicly subsidized. If the Pharmaceutical Benefits Advisory Committee (PBAC), an independent government advisory body, decides against including a product in the public drug program, the drug's manufacturers can now demand a review of the procedure.

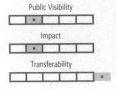

In Australia, newly registered prescription drugs are subsidized through the Pharmaceutical Benefits Scheme only if they are listed on the Pharmaceutical Benefits Schedule. Manufacturers usually apply to the PBAC. The applications take the form of detailed, evidence-based reports on the effectiveness and cost-effectiveness of the drug in comparison to alternative treatment options. The evidence should justify the price the manufacturer is asking for the drug. The government-appointed PBAC has 10 members, who are physicians, pharmacologists, economists, pharmacists and representatives of the consumers' associations. They are in turn advised by economists, epidemiologists and statisticians.

New pharmaceuticals are listed on the basis of effectiveness and cost-effectiveness

Only drugs that have received a positive recommendation from

PBAC recommen-
dations are
binding

the PBAC can be placed on the list of drugs entitled to subsidies by the Ministry of Health. In a second step, the Pharmaceutical Benefits Pricing Authority, a state body acting on the recommendations of the PBAC, decides on a suitable price to offer the manufacturer, and the Ministry of Health negotiates with the manufacturer on this basis. In Australia, therefore, the assessment by the PBAC is the most important basis for the reimbursement and the regulation of prices of newly registered drugs.

Reviews can now
be requested

The new feature of this process, introduced in February 2005, is that the manufacturer, including U.S. companies, can now request a review if the PBAC has reached a negative recommendation. In the bilateral free trade agreement AUFSTA, which came into force at the beginning of January 2005, Australia undertook to make the system of drug regulation more transparent and to involve the pharmaceutical industry more in the process of evaluation of its products.

If the manufacturer lodges an objection to the recommendation of the PBAC, then under the review mechanism a convenor will appoint a reviewer from a panel of independent experts. On the basis of the evidence submitted, the reviewer can clarify controversial issues with the manufacturers, the PBAC or the Ministry and reevaluate the evidence; however, the reviewer is not allowed to take new information into account. The PBAC must then decide whether the conclusions of the reviewer's report warrant an alteration of its own recommendation. It must explain its decision in a report to the Ministry and Minister.

More accountabil-
ity and transpar-
ency

The PBAC has faced criticism from some producer organizations and manufacturers about the lack of transparency in its decision-making, although in the past this has been driven by commercial-in-confidence issues imposed by manufacturers themselves. There have been some moves towards greater transparency and since 2003, it has published all negative decisions, including the reasons advanced. In the reformed evaluation procedure now agreed on, it will have to publish all review reports.

Potential conflicts
ahead

It remains unclear what will happen if the PBAC's final recommendation and the reviewer's report conflict. In this situation, it would be up to the Ministry to reach a decision on the basis of scientific opinions that contradict one another. Political considerations would then play a greater role. The health minister has already overridden the most important advisory body in the Australian pharmaceuticals sector once in the past. Despite a negative recommendation from the PBAC in 2001, the government approved subsidies for a drug for breast cancer by agreeing to provide the funding through channels outside the PBS program. It remains to be seen whether the PBAC will find its authority undermined by the new Australian review procedures for the evaluation of pharmaceutical products. In the event of conflicts, and under pressure from manufacturers, the Ministry could find it easier to override the PBAC and publicity fund pharmaceuticals outside the PBS using the alternative described here.

Sources and further reading:
Abbott, Tony. Australia-United States Free Trade Agreement and the Pharmaceutical Benefit Scheme. February 4, 2005. www.health.gov.au/internet/wcms/publishing.nsf/Content/health-mediarel-yr2005 -ta-abb00 8.htm.
Burton, Kate, and Jacob Varghese. The PBS and the Australia-US Free Trade Agreement. Research Note 2004-05 No. 3, July 21, 2004, Parliamentary Library. www.aph.gov.au/library/pubs/rn/2004-05/05rn03.pdf.
Department of Foreign Affairs and Trade. Australia-United States Free Trade Agreement, Chapter 2, Annex 2C. www.dfat.gov.au/trade/negotiations/us_fta/final-text/chapter_2.html.
Department of Foreign Affairs and Trade. Australia-United States Free Trade Agreement—Fact Sheets. www.dfat.gov.au/trade/negotiations/us_fta/outcomes/index.html.
Joint Parliamentary Committee on Treaties. Report Number 61: Australia-United States Free Trade Agreement. www.aph.gov.au/house/committee/jsct/usafta/report.htm.

United States: Preferred drug lists

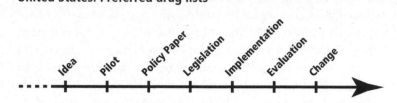

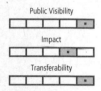

Public Visibility

Impact

Transferability

Over the past two years, about 20 of the U.S. states have introduced lists of drugs that physicians should prefer when writing prescriptions for patients under Medicaid. With this so-called "preferred drug list," states such as Florida, Georgia, Illinois, Kentucky, Louisiana, Maryland, Michigan and Oregon aim to reduce the state expenditure on pharmaceutical products while at the same time promoting the use of therapeutically beneficial products. The inclusion of a drug on the lists is based on scientific evidence regarding its effectiveness, safety and costs in comparison with other products in the same therapeutic class.

Rising expenditure on drugs

Medicaid's constantly increasing spending on pharmaceuticals is one of the most important financial burdens the states face. This is made more acute by the poor state of the economy, with growing numbers of lower-income earners entitled to insurance under the system. Throughout the United States, public spending on prescription drugs rose from some $40 billion (€33 billion) in 1990 to $140 billion (€115 billion) in 2001, which represents an increase of 250 percent. In 2001, Medicaid alone spent $24 billion (€20 billion) on prescription drugs, which accounted for 11 percent of its entire health care expenditure.

Preferred drug lists

In the hope of promoting high-quality pharmaceuticals that are also favorably priced, preferred drug lists have become a favorite and widespread instrument in health policies in the United States. These are not positive lists in the strict sense of the term: Under the national framework legislation for the Medicaid program, the states cannot completely exclude a specific drug from public reimbursement. Instead, many states place administrative barriers in the way of physicians and patients in the case of unlisted products.

Approved exceptions

Physicians in Michigan, for example, must first obtain the approval of the Medicaid authority before they can prescribe a

74

medicine that is not listed; in Oregon, they have to state explicitly on the prescription that the patient should receive a product not included on the list. Pharmacists are reimbursed for nonlisted drugs only if they are approved exceptions. Pharmaceutical manufacturers can improve the probability that their product will be selected for listing from a number of similarly effective medicines by offering Medicaid a rebate on the price of the drug and thus reducing the cost for the treatment.

At first, the initiators of the preferred drug lists—government and Medicaid authorities—met with considerable opposition from the pharmaceutical industry, health care providers and patient groups, who were opposed to the higher barriers against nonlisted pharmaceutical products and felt that appropriate patient care would be threatened.

Initial resistance ...

In many states, the manufacturers went to court against the introduction of the preferred drug lists, but in a precedence case in 2003 in Michigan these were declared compatible with federal law, as were the manufacturer's rebates and the approval procedures for nonlisted products.

Meanwhile, however, most pharmaceutical manufacturers have decided to cooperate, because they can increase the market share of their products if they provide them for Medicaid at more favorable prices than the equivalent products of their competitors, and are therefore included on the list.

... gives way to calculated cooperation

The fact that the decision to introduce the preferred drug lists was expressly based on scientific evidence helped to overcome the skepticism of physicians and patients in the long term. The experience in the United States shows that over time, the initially controversial evidence-based drug lists have met with the acceptance of most interest groups.

Sources and further reading:
Center for Evidence-Based Policy, Drug Effectiveness Review Project: www.ohsu.edu/drugeffectiveness/description/index.htm
Bernasek, Cathy, Catherine Harrington, Dan Mendelson, and Ryan Padrex. Oregon's Medicaid PDL: Will an Evidence-Based Formulary with Voluntary Compliance Set

a Precedent for Medicaid? Henry J. Kaiser Family Foundation 2003. www.kff.org/medicaid/4173.cfm.

Centers for Medicare and Medicaid Services Office. National Health Accounts. Health Expenditure Projections 2002--2012. www.cms.hhs.gov/statistics/nhe.

Crowley, Jeffrey S., Deb Ashner, and Linda Elam. Medicaid Outpatient Prescription Drug Benefits: Findings from a National Survey. Kaiser Commission on Medicaid and the Uninsured 2003. www.kff.org/medicaid/4164.cfm.

Kaye, Neva. Affording Prescription Drugs: State Initiatives to Contain Cost and Improve Access. National Academy for State Health Policy 2002. www.nashp.org/_docdisp_page.cfm?LID=666CB5DC-7948-11D6-BD1700A0CC76FF4C.

Neumann, Peter. Evidence-Based and Value-Based Formulary Guidelines. *Health Affairs* (23) 1 2004: 124–134.

Finland: Expensive drugs for rare diseases

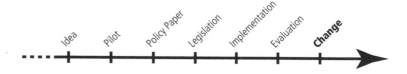

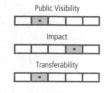

Public Visibility

Impact

Transferability

Simplified approval for "orphan drugs"

In February 2005, the parliamentary ombudsman of Finland declared that hospitals would be acting illegally if they refused to treat a patient with Fabry's syndrome due to the high cost of the drugs required.

In 2001, the European Agency for the Evaluation of Medicinal Products approved for the first time drugs for a series of genetic enzyme deficiency disorders that had previously been untreatable (Fabry's syndrome, Gaucher's syndrome, and MPS 1 disorders). The accelerated central market certification procedure places less severe criteria on the proof of efficacy for so-called "orphan drugs" than for other drugs. The aim is to make drugs for the treatment of rare disorders with a prevalence of less than

5/10,000 available to patients more quickly and to promote research into orphan drugs.

The few placebo-controlled studies of enzyme replacement therapy of lysosomal storage disorders, which were carried out exclusively by the pharmaceutical manufacturers themselves, showed some benefits, such as less pain, improved kidney function and a decline in the storage products in the organs typical of these disorders. But in most cases, nothing was known about long-term effects.

Scant evidence about long-term effects

This lack of convincing evidence is a serious problem for those who have to meet the costs of treatment, namely the Finnish municipalities and hospital districts. For example, the lifelong stationary enzyme substitution by means of infusions to treat Fabry's syndrome, which affects some 30 patients in Finland, costs €200,000 to €300,000 per patient each year.

Within the framework of a study, the drug manufacturers provided 13 Fabry patients with the therapy without charge for two years. After the conclusion of the study in 2004, however, many hospitals refused to provide the treatment, arguing that the costs were too high in view of the unclear long-term effects of the treatment. Municipalities tried without success to pass responsibility for the funding on to the government in Helsinki.

Public pressure

Supported by pharmaceutical companies, the Finnish Fabry Society then lodged a complaint with the parliamentary ombudsman, Riitta-Leena Paunio. One of the Society's arguments was that the cost for enzyme replacement therapy was being met in many other European countries.

The ombudsman is responsible for examining public measures impartially and preventing the unfair treatment of specific groups. In this case, she judged that the Finnish Fabry patients are legally entitled to enzyme replacement therapy because, as she explained at the beginning of the year, prioritization decisions must not lead to necessary treatment being refused on the grounds of the costs involved. They should take into consideration only the needs of the patient, the nature of the disorder and the effectiveness of the treatment. In her opinion, the legislation would have to be amended before economic aspects could also be taken into account.

Incurable diseases can be costly

Experts, on the other hand, emphasize that it is usual and also

justified in Finland to take the costs of treatments into consideration in relation to their effectiveness. As a consequence of the
statement of the parliamentary ombudsman, some hospitals
districts have now once again begun to offer the expensive treatment for Fabry patients.

It is still unclear whether the statement by Riitta-Leena Paunio
will also have an effect on the relative weight of effectiveness and
cost-effectiveness in prioritization decisions in the case of other
diseases. Since it is to be expected that an increasing number of
expensive pharmaceutical drugs will be developed for small
populations of patients, Finland will now have to consider very
carefully how to resolve the contradictions between the law and
the practical realities.

> *Sources and further reading:*
> Parliamentary Ombudsman: *www.oikeusasiamies.fi/Resource*
> *.phx/eoa/english/index.htx*

Spain: Pharmaceutical reform in decentralized health care system

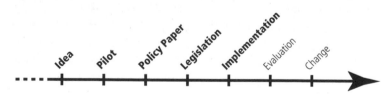

Public Visibility

Impact

Transferability

By the end of 2006, the Spanish central government hopes to
have saved €300 million in the public health care sector by means
of a comprehensive drug reform package, which should also ensure that pharmaceutical products are prescribed and used more
rationally. The 67 individual provisions in the program, published
by the Minister for Health and Consumer Protection in November 2004, address the key problems in the Spanish pharmaceutical sector.

Improved access,
...

Firstly, the process of drug licensing is to be accelerated; in
addition, an evaluation committee is to be set up to provide a
scientific assessment of the added therapeutic benefits offered by

new products. Drugs offering significant advantages over existing products are to be made available without any significant delay and included in the benefit basket. The Spanish Ministry of Health has announced that it will issue a positive list this year.

The program is also intended to promote the quality of medication. The government is planning to promote projects and studies that systematically identify the undesirable effects of drug therapies and help to prevent these. The intention is to initiate a debate on the pros and cons of commercial versus independent drug information for patients and prescribing physicians, as well as to advance models for electronic prescriptions. However, hardly any details are available as yet.

... better quality, ...

The government's main objective is to intervene in the distribution of drugs and the regulation of prices so as to slow down the rise in expenditure for pharmaceuticals. The profit margins of pharmacists were lowered this year from 9.6 to 8.6 percent. In 2006, they are to fall by a further percentage point. Secondly, the pharmaceutical manufacturers were obliged to provide a rebate of 2 percent on public sales, against their vehement resistance. The drug companies regard this as an unconstitutional additional tax, even though the government announced that the rebates would be lower for companies that spent more on research and development. The drug companies had to lower the retail prices of pharmaceuticals this year by 4.2 percent, and there will be a further reduction of 2 percent in March 2006—unless the product was approved within the previous year or subject to the reference pricing system.

... lower costs

The reference pricing system is at the heart of the current debate on drug policies in Spain. As an element of their program on pharmaceuticals for 2007, the Socialist government has announced a comprehensive reform of the system, but it gave no more details about what this would entail. It only established that there would be no further changes to the current system until the reform was implemented. That means that in the next two years there will not be any modification of the levels of the reference price, nor will any new products that are now out of patent be included in the system.

Dissatisfaction in the regions and the drug industry

This temporary termination of the reference pricing system, which was introduced in 2000 under the Conservative government as one of the major innovations of Spanish drug policies over the past 10 years (see issue 2 of "Health Policy Developments"), has received sharp criticism from the Spanish regional governments. They object that companies whose products lose patent protection in the transition period are artificially and unjustifiably excluded from the reference pricing system—to the disadvantage of the regions (as the payers), the patients and the manufacturers of generics.

The PSOE government is above all accused of not integrating the regional governments sufficiently in the formulation of the central reform strategy, although in the end they will bear responsibility for funding the pharmaceuticals. Regions under the control of the conservative Partido Popular in particular see this as an attempt by Madrid, despite decentralization of the Spanish health system completed in 2002 (see issue 3 of "Health Policy Developments"), to retain control in certain areas of health policy and to prepare the way for recentralization.

The pharmaceutical companies, on the other hand, complain that the planned reference pricing reform, in combination with the additional evaluation procedure for new drugs (the details of which have also not yet been specified), will only serve to create uncertainty among both manufacturers and consumers.

Unclear criteria   It is true that the Ministry of Health has not yet explained the criteria by which drugs will in future be categorized in a reference price group. Farmaindustria, the most important Spanish pharmaceutical association, gave advance warning that the existing equivalence criteria for drugs should not be changed at all. In Spain, these take into account only the chemical structure, not the pharmacological or therapeutic comparability, as in Germany, for example.

It will also be necessary to define the criteria and methods by which the additional benefits of new drugs are to be evaluated, as well as whether the evaluation of cost-effectiveness should be an element of the new evaluation procedure and whether the evaluation should be integrated with the reform of the reference pricing system (and if so, how).

Experts generally agree that there is a need in Spain for a broad review of health policies with the aim of providing better and less expensive medication, and that—in theory—the proposals of the Ministry of Health would represent such a step forward. But so far a large part of the program has not been worked out in detail, nor has it been approved by parliament, not to mention the need to reach the necessary consensus with the regional governments.

Sources and further reading:

Ministerio de Sanidad y Consumo. Plan Estratégico de Política Farmacéutica para el Sistema Nacional de Salud. November 2004 .

Ministerio de Sanidad y Consumo. Real Decreto 2402/2004, de 30 de diciembre, por el que se desarrolla el artículo 104 de la Ley 25/1990, de 20 de diciembre, del Medicamento, para las revisiones coyunturales de precios de especialidades farmacéuticas y se adoptan medidas adicionales para la contención del gasto farmacéutico. Boletín Oficial del Estado 31 December 2004.

Consejo de Estado. Dictamen del Consejo de Estado sobre el proyecto de Real decreto que desarrolla el artículo 104 de la Ley 25/1990, del Medicamento, y que suspende los precios de referencia.

Newsflash

Israel: End-of-life care policy

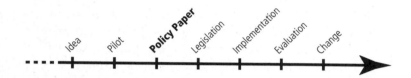

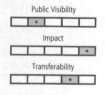

Expert committee for palliative care

Inadequate provisions for hospices and specialist caregivers

A professional committee appointed by the Director-General of the Ministry of Health recommended that comprehensive palliative care should be provided to all terminally ill patients and their families. The Director-General expressed a strong commitment to the recommendations presented to him in April 2005.

With this step, the ministry is following the recommendations of a committee it had appointed, made up of primary care physicians and specialists, nurses, social workers, scientists, representatives of the health plans and nongovernmental organizations. At the start of the year, the experts for palliative care had presented a report in which they formulated the objectives of ensuring that all people in need should be provided with palliative care at the end of their life and improving the quality of life of the patients and their next of kin.

Palliative care, developed during the last decades of the 20th century, is now regarded as "state of the art" in the care of the terminally ill. But Israeli studies point out that, as in other countries, numerous obstacles stand in the way of its implementation. These barriers include the social and professional taboos regarding dying and death, as well as system-related obstacles.

In Israel, some 2,000 people each year receive palliative care in the final stages of an incurable illness, but in the opinion of experts this corresponds to less than 10 percent of the patients in need. In the country as a whole, there are three hospices and seven outpatient palliative care facilities run by the health plans, nongovernmental organizations or hospitals, and these are for the most part funded by donations.

The care for the terminally ill is usually provided by dedicated individuals who are convinced of the necessity and importance of all-around care in a hospice setting. In hospitals or cancer centers, on the other hand, the emphasis is often primarily on the control of physical symptoms, such as pain. Less importance is attached to the psychosocial and spiritual care also demanded by the WHO.

Medical specialists and advocates of palliative care have complained for some time about shortcomings in Israel in terms of qualifications, structures and resources. As in many other countries, the health care system is not prepared for the aging population and the growing numbers of chronically ill patients, although this fact has meanwhile been recognized by politicians and the general public. Palliative care became a topic of political debate recently in the course of the passage through the Knesset of a "Dying Patients Law," which, as in Australia, Belgium, France, the Netherlands and Switzerland, allows for passive euthanasia— withholding life-prolonging measures from the terminally ill.

The professional committee proposed that palliative care will be offered for terminally ill patients with incurable cancer, congestive heart failure, chronic obstructive pulmonary disease, renal failure, AIDS, dementia, degenerative neurological diseases (e.g., amyotrophic lateral sclerosis) or coma. A detailed assessment defines the care the individual needs. The wishes of the patients and their families, for example regarding the degree of sedation, should be taken into account.

Who receives palliative services?

Two physicians must first assess that the patient has less than six months left to live. Some criticize this provision, because studies suggest that the remaining survival period is only estimated correctly in about one third of cases. Furthermore, the definition goes against the modern concept of palliative care, which attempts to combine curative and palliative care from the beginning of a progressive illness.

Providing further training

The program outlines plans for palliative care on two levels: by family physicians, internists, geriatric oncologists, pediatricians and caregivers on the primary level and by palliative care specialists on the secondary level. The latter will also be responsible for providing information, specialist support and further training for the primary care providers. Every hospital and every outpatient clinic will have a specialized palliative team of physicians and caregivers. Training in palliative care will be increased, both for primary care providers and specialists.

The committee proposed that patients would be given choice between palliative care at home, in hospital or in a care institution. Care institutions are to be made available every day around the clock and accessible throughout the country. The recommendation of the committee call for increasing the number of palliative beds—for example by reassigning beds from other specialties—from about 80 to 300, that is, 12 to 45 beds per million inhabitants.

Costs increasing or falling?

There is disagreement about funding the program. The four major Israeli health plans oppose the view of the Ministry of Health and Ministry of Finance that health costs will fall with improved palliative care. Even if costs for hospital stays are decreased, experts expect that the Israeli strategy for palliative care can succeed only if additional financial resources are provided, primarily for the outpatient sector.

Sources and further reading:
Bentur, Netta, Shirli Resnitzky, and Yitshak Shnoor. Palliative Care in the Israeli Health Care System. Jerusalem: Myers-JDC-Brookdale Institute, 2005 (in Hebrew).
Emanuel, Ezekiel J. Cost savings at the end of life. What do the data show? *Journal of the American Medical Association* (275) 1996: 1907–1914.
Hughes, Susan L., Alec Ulasevich, Frances M. Weaver, William Henderson, Larry Manheim, Joseph D. Kubal, and Frank Bonarigo. Impact of home care on hospital days: A meta-analysis. *Health Services Research* (32) 1997: 415–432.
Morrison, R. Sean, and Diane E. Meier. Palliative care. *New England Journal of Medicine* (350) 2004: 2582–2590.

Smith, Thomas. Adding hospice and palliative care services to the cancer center menu. *Journal of Palliative Medicine* (6) 2003: 641–644.

The SUPPORT principal investigators. Controlled trial to improve care for seriously ill hospitalized patients. The study to understand prognoses and preferences for outcomes and risk of treatment (SUPPORT). *Journal of the American Medical Association* (274) 1995: 1591-1598.

Singapore: Internet transparency reduces hospital bills

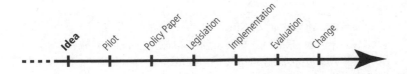

With improved transparency on hospital bills, the Ministry of Health in Singapore has managed to increase competition between hospitals and has achieved price reductions for inpatient services.

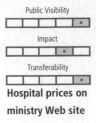

Hospital prices on ministry Web site

Since the end of 2003, the ministry Web site has provided information about the median values of the prices that hospitals charge their patients for 70 common medical diagnoses and procedures.

All 26 public and private hospitals, and specialist centers as well, were obliged to make invoicing data available—a measure that led to an immediate and continuing downward trend in hospital fees. Prices fell for gallbladder removal, for tonsillectomy and for treating pneumonia and strokes. The greatest reduction came in the case of laser surgery to correct nearsightedness: In the two leading hospitals, the price plummeted by 40 percent within ten months. Managers from hospitals with higher charges found that they had to either provide a justification for the prices or reduce them. The price comparison also showed that for the same diagnosis or procedure, the private hospitals were charging between 20 and 120 percent more.

Transparency reduces prices

Half the hospitals and clinics in Singapore are public institutions, providing 11,798 beds, that is, 80 percent of all beds. Like the private hospitals, they determine the prices for medical treatments and procedures on their own. The government only regulates the charge for the so-called hotel component, depending on the levels of catering and accommodation provided. The consequence is lively competition to attract patients among the city-state's four million inhabitants and from neighboring countries.

Positive public reaction

In the past, cost indicators were not particularly transparent, so the public has welcomed the Internet price comparisons and the resulting reductions in hospital charges. At the same time, the move has left the public pondering how the hospitals managed to get away with charging inflated prices for so long.

> *Sources and further reading:*
> Ministry of Health, Hospital Bill Size: *www.moh.gov.sg/corp/charges/common/procedures.do*

Finland: Research in primary care centers

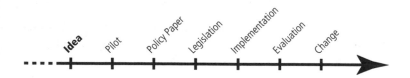

Public Visibility

Impact

Transferability

Research in primary care underdeveloped

The Finnish Minister of Health would like to see more research work carried out in the primary health care centers of the 450 municipalities in the country.

In Finland, most of the funding the government and the National Research Council provide for health research goes to university hospitals. But when it comes to formulating health policies aimed at the further development of primary care, their findings are of little assistance. Scientific projects are rare in the primary care sector itself, and the training programs for primary care physicians interested in research are underdeveloped. This is one of the main motives for the change in policy announced by the health minister, who is herself a public health expert and dentist.

She draws on an a report commissioned by the Ministry of Social Affairs and Health, published at the start of the year, that analyzes the current state of research activities in primary care in Finland. The experts conducted a survey of research workers and physicians in health care centers and universities, and also provided a review of scientific publications covering strategies adopted in other countries for research in the primary care sector. The authors made a series of recommendations about the promotion of research and scientific training in Finland's primary care sector.

In close cooperation with universities, projects are to be developed that are relevant for public health and address prevention, quality, effectiveness, and cost-effectiveness of diagnosis and therapy, as well as rehabilitation services and the organizational structures of primary care. Research teams in the primary care centers will receive further training from academic faculties, which will also provide supervision. The public health experts' report recommends that the research activities and their results be monitored and evaluated continuously and be made transparent by means of an open-access database. **Cooperation with academic institutions**

The primary health care centers, which are organized and maintained by the municipalities, provide a range of services including primary medical care, dental care, and mother and child care, as well as preventive and health-promoting services. Many health centers suffer from staffing problems, and in particular from a shortage of physicians. It is thought that primary care could be made more attractive if scientific work and practical work could be better combined in future, with periods of research and scientific training alternating with practical clinic work. **Primary health care centers as attractive workplaces**

Currently, the Ministry of Health is consulting with other ministries, government agencies, municipalities, professional associations, universities, and the Research Council about the program and the legal and financial changes that will be necessary. It will be interesting to see the stances adopted by the interested groups, such as the universities and municipalities. The Minister of Health has announced plans to finance research in the primary care sector by siphoning off tax funding currently going to uni- **Ongoing consultations** versity research. Certainly the prospects of a successful outcome of the annual negotiations with the Ministry of Finance for the new health budget seem greater if the Ministry of Social Affairs and Health shows it will not be requiring any additional input of resources.

Sources and further reading:
Mattila, Jukka, and Marjukka Mäkelä. Research in health centers: Present state and future. Working Group Memoranda of the Ministry of Social Affairs and Health. Helsinki 2005. www.stm.fi/Resource.phx/publishing/store/2005/03/pr1109252784945/passthru.pdf (in Finnish), www.stm.fi/Resource.phx/publishing/documents/3120/summary_en.htx (English summary).

Reform Tracker

Country, *Chapter*, Title, Issue, Page

Australia

Funding and Reimbursement
Private health insurance incentive scheme; I, 22

Integration of Care/Coordination of Care
Coordinated care trials; III, 29
General practitioners' remuneration; IV, 48

Health and Aging
National Strategy for an Ageing Australia; II, 24

Human Resources for Health
Policy responses to chronic and acute shortages in the
nursing workforce; II, 67

Mental Health
Beyond Blue—National depression initiative; IV, 21

Patient Safety
HealthConnect; V, 41

Pharmaceutical Policies
Drug evaluation and free trade agreement with the United
States; V, 71

Primary Care
Primary Care Collaboratives; III, 28

Public Health and Prevention
Optimizing cancer management: The New South Wales
Cancer Institute; II, 86 (Newsflash)

Austria

Advancing Health Care Organization
Health Reform 2005; IV, 68

Funding and Reimbursement
Adjustment of health insurance contribution rates; I, 20

Health and Aging
Family Hospice Sabbatical; II, 32
Ten years of LTC coverage; II, 39

Pharmaceutical Policies
Criteria for reimbursable drugs and promotion of generics;
II, 57

(Re-)Centralization versus Decentralization
Health purchasing agencies; III, 46

Canada

Access
Is the Health Care Guarantee losing ground? IV, 37

Accountability and Participation
Independent health policy advice; III, 23

Human Resources for Health
A co-coordinated and comprehensive approach to health
human resource planning; II, 73

Integration of Care/Coordination of Care
Public insurance to cover post-acute home care; I, 47
Primary care reform; III, 33

Patient Safety
Institute for Patient Safety, V; 37

Quality Management
Barcelona and Montreal compare their health care services;
IV, 61
Independent council for quality improvement; I, 37
Independent council for quality improvement in health
care; II, 85 (Newsflash)

Denmark

Access
No-show fees for nonattending patients; IV, 39

Accountability and Participation
An open and transparent health care system; III, 22

Funding and Reimbursement
The search for the right mix of roles; I, 31

Health and Aging
Free choice of provider of personal and practical help; II,
31

Pharmaceutical Policies
Emphasis on economic evaluation of new pharmaceuticals;
II, 56

Public Health and Prevention
Denmark: More signs instead of less smoke; V, 66

(Re-)Centralization versus Decentralization
Strategy for the health care system—The patient; III, 44
Public sector reform and hospital management—A political agreement; IV, 79 (Newsflash)

Technical Innovations and Bioethics
Electronic patient records in hospitals; III, 53

Finland

Access
Supplementary outpatient fees; IV, 36

Accountability and Participation
Vouchers in social and health care; III, 24

Funding and Reimbursement
Plans to reform the hospital billing system; I, 32

Pharmaceutical Policies
Generic substitution of prescription drugs; II, 59
New Development Center for Drug Therapy; II, 60
Restricting generic substitution; IV, 77 (Newsflash)
Finland: Expensive drugs for rare diseases; V, 76

Primary Care
Finland: Research in primary care centers (Newsflash); V, 86

Public Health and Prevention
Finland: Major reduction in alcohol tax; V, 59

Quality Management
The debate about the right level of specialized care; I, 40

(Re-)Centralization versus Decentralization
County-level management of welfare services; III, 44

France

Access
Health insurance vouchers plan; IV, 29
Health Insurance Reform; II, 76 (Newsflash)
High Council on the future of sickness insurance; III, 67
(Newsflash)

Funding and Reimbursement
Hôpital 2007; V, 27
Ambulatory care system caught between physicians and
private insurance; V, 30

Health and Aging
Towards long-term care reform; II, 35

Integration of Care/Coordination of Care
Toward a nursing care plan for the disabled; I, 48

Pharmaceutical Policies
Lower reimbursement rates and delisting of pharmaceu-
ticals; II, 50
Liberalization of prices for innovative medicines; II, 52

Primary Care
Improved coordination in health care; IV, 47

Public Health and Prevention
Draft five-year public health plan; I, 53
Reform of the public health law; III, 40
Ambitious public health policy threatened, V, 45

Technical Innovations and Bioethics
Bioethics legislation; III, 55

Germany

Funding and Reimbursement
Co-payments for outpatient care, V; 22

Health and Aging
Proposals to achieve financial sustainability of LTCI; II, 40

Integration of Care/Coordination of Care
Disease Management Programs combine quality and financial incentives; III, 32

Primary Care
Family doctors as gatekeepers; IV, 52

Quality Management
Plans for a "Center for Quality in Medicine"; I, 38
Compulsory external quality assurance for hospitals; IV, 56

Israel

Access
Co-payments, access, equity; IV, 30

Advancing Health Care Organization
For-profit sickness fund; IV, 65

Primary Care
Improvement of primary care quality; IV, 51

Public Health and Prevention
Health plans assume responsibility for preventive care; V, 47

Health and Aging
End-of-life care policy; V, 82 (Newsflash)

Japan

Advancing Health Care Organization
Plan for merger of insurers; IV, 73

Funding and Reimbursement
Increase of co-payment rates; I, 21

Public Health and Prevention
Striving for "Healthy Japan 21"; III, 41
Ban on blood donations against variant Creutzfeldt-Jakob
disease; V, 53

New Zealand

Funding and Reimbursement
Prepaid general practice fee; I, 22

Health and Aging
Removal of assets test for older people in long-term resi-
dential care; II, 42

Human Resources for Health
Workforce development; II, 72

Mental Health
A national mental health plan; IV, 23

Pharmaceutical Policies
Direct-to-consumer advertising of prescription medicines;
II, 66

Public Health and Prevention
Cancer control action plan, V, 49
100 percent smoke-free, V, 64

Primary Care
Care Plus for high-needs patients; IV, 45
Primary Health Organizations; I, 55

Quality Management
Improving quality—A strategic approach; II, 87 (News-flash)

(Re-)Centralization versus Decentralization
Interim evaluation of District Health Boards; III, 50

Netherlands

Accountability and Participation
Client-linked personal budgets; III, 25

Advancing Health Care Organization
New health insurance system; IV, 66
Social Support Act (WMO); IV, 80 (Newsflash)

Funding and Reimbursement
Rationing benefits; I, 24

Health and Aging
Compulsory health insurance (AWBZ) and long-term care; II, 26
Integrated care for the elderly; II, 27
Human Resources for Health

Coping with prospective shortages in the medical work-force; II, 70

Quality Management
Compulsory quality improvement; I, 42
Quality management more compulsory; II, 84 (Newsflash)

Singapore

South Korea

Spain

Access
Facilitating specialized services and medication for illegal immigrants; IV, 33

Health and Aging
Second plan for integrating health and social care in Castilla y Léon; II, 28
Toledo Agreement and LTC insurance; II, 33

Integration of Care/Coordination of Care
A pilot project for integrated care in Catalonia; I, 50

Pharmaceutical Policies
Reference pricing system for generic medicines: Update and extension; II, 62
Pharmaceutical reform in decentralized health care system; V, 78

Public Health and Prevention
Weak anti-tobacco law, V, 61

Quality Management
Barcelona and Montreal compare their health care services; IV, 61
National Health System Act—The debate about decentralization, cohesion and quality of care; I, 43

(Re-)Centralization versus Decentralization
Evaluating regional health care financing; III, 49

Technical Innovations and Bioethics
Electronic drug management; III, 54

Switzerland

Advancing Health Care Organization
Relaunching integrated networks of care; IV, 70

Emerging Issues
Health impact assessment of Ticino's public policy; IV, 24

Funding and Reimbursement
Failed referendum proposal to remove per-capita premium
health insurance; I, 28
Individual passage of the reforms of the health insurance
act; III, 63 (Newsflash)
A drop of solidarity in the ocean of inequality; V, 18

Health and Aging
Long-term care insurance not (yet) in sight; II, 37

(Re-)Centralization versus Decentralization
Improving territorial equity in a federal state; III, 47

United Kingdom

Access
United Kingdom: Knights, knaves and gnashers; IV, 40

Accountability and Participation
England: Choice and responsiveness in the English
National Health Service; III, 20

Funding and Reimbursement
England: Alternative methods of health care financing; I,
29
England: Role of the private sector; I, 30
England: NHS Foundation Trusts; I, 34

Hawaii: New legislative move toward universal health insurance; I, 64
Oregon: Oregon Health Plan cuts; III, 60 (Newsflash)
United States: Proposal for Medicaid Reform; I, 58
United States: Proposal for SCHIP Reform; I, 59
United States: Presidential candidates' proposals for health insurance; II, 80 (Newsflash)
United States: Health Insurance Portability and Accountability Act of 1996; II, 83 (Newsflash)

Funding and Reimbursement
United States: Tax credits for the uninsured to purchase health insurance; I, 61
United States: Individual mandate for health insurance; V, 16

Health and Aging
United States: Expansion of prescription drug coverage for the elderly; II, 45

Human Resources for Health
California: First-in-nation rules on nurse-to-patient ratios; II, 67

Patient Safety
United States: Patient Safety and Quality Improvement Act; V, 34
United States: Hospital Compare; V, 39

Pharmaceutical Policies
California: Prescription drug reimportation legislation; III, 62 (Newsflash)
California: Prescription Drug Reimportation Bill; IV, 75 (Newsflash)
United States: Preferred drug lists; V, 74

Public Health and Prevention
California: Obesity Prevention Initiative; V, 56
United States: Ban on soft drinks in schools; III, 37